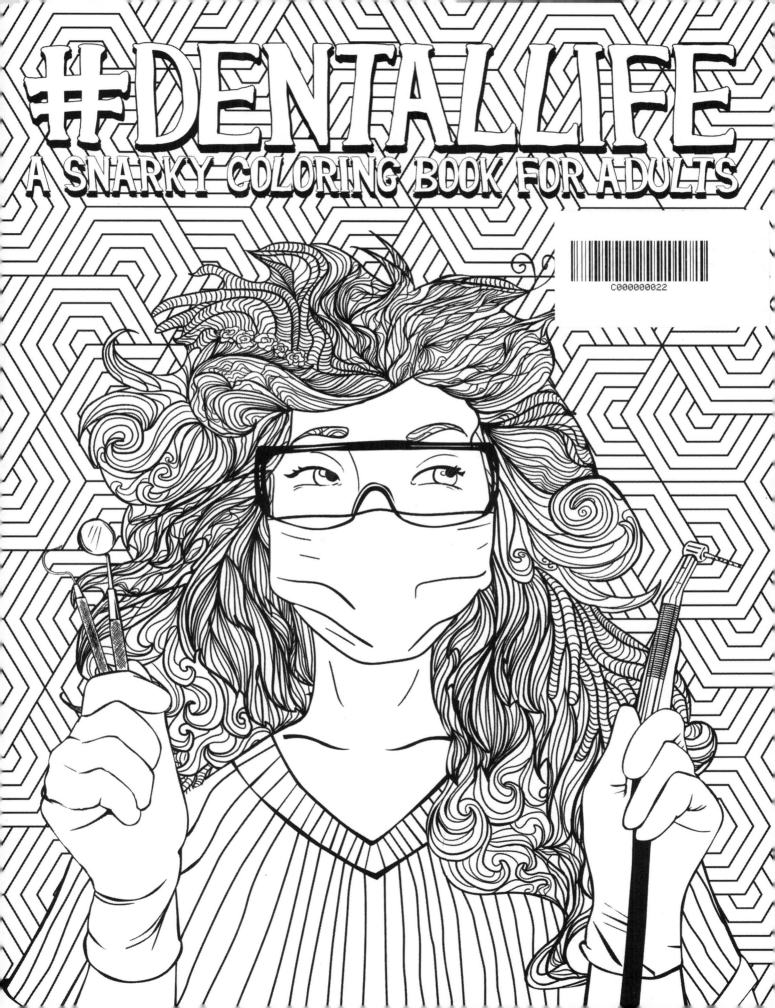

Want free goodies?
Email us at freebies@pbleu.com

@papeteriebleu

Papeterie Bleu

Shop our other books at
www.pbleu.com

Wholesale distribution through Ingram Content Group
www.ingramcontent.com/publishers/distribution/wholesale

For questions and customer service, email us at
support@pbleu.com

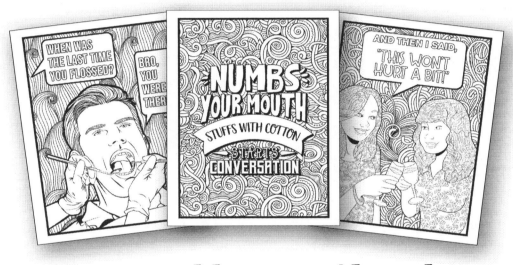
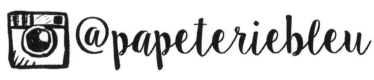
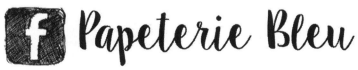

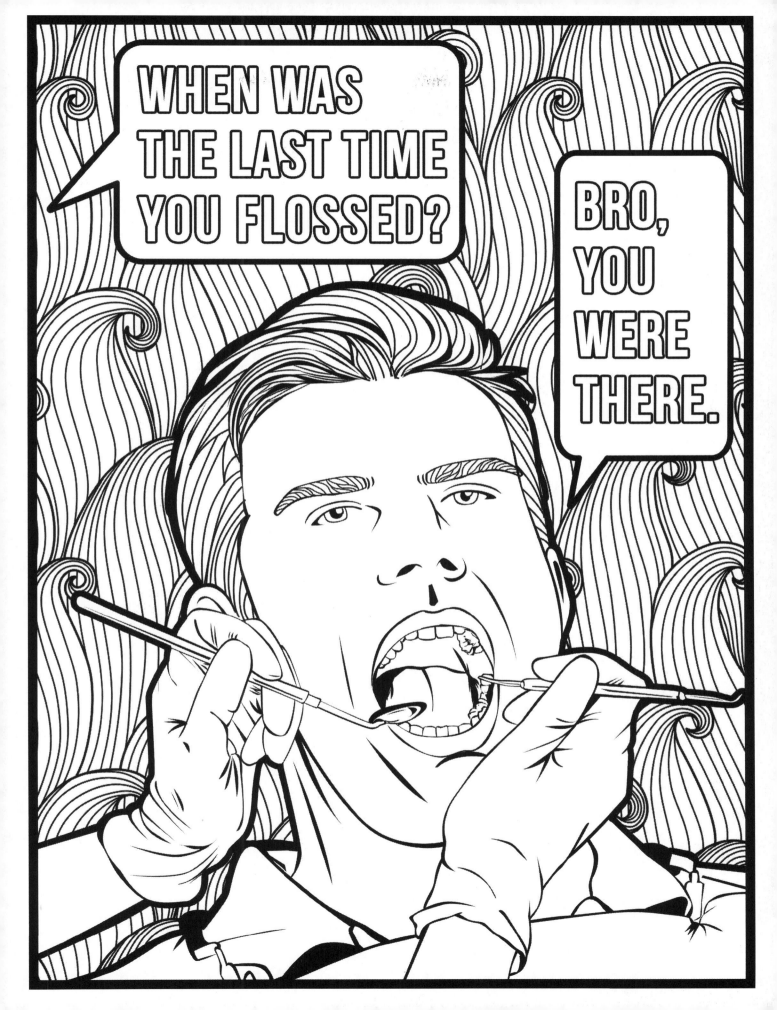

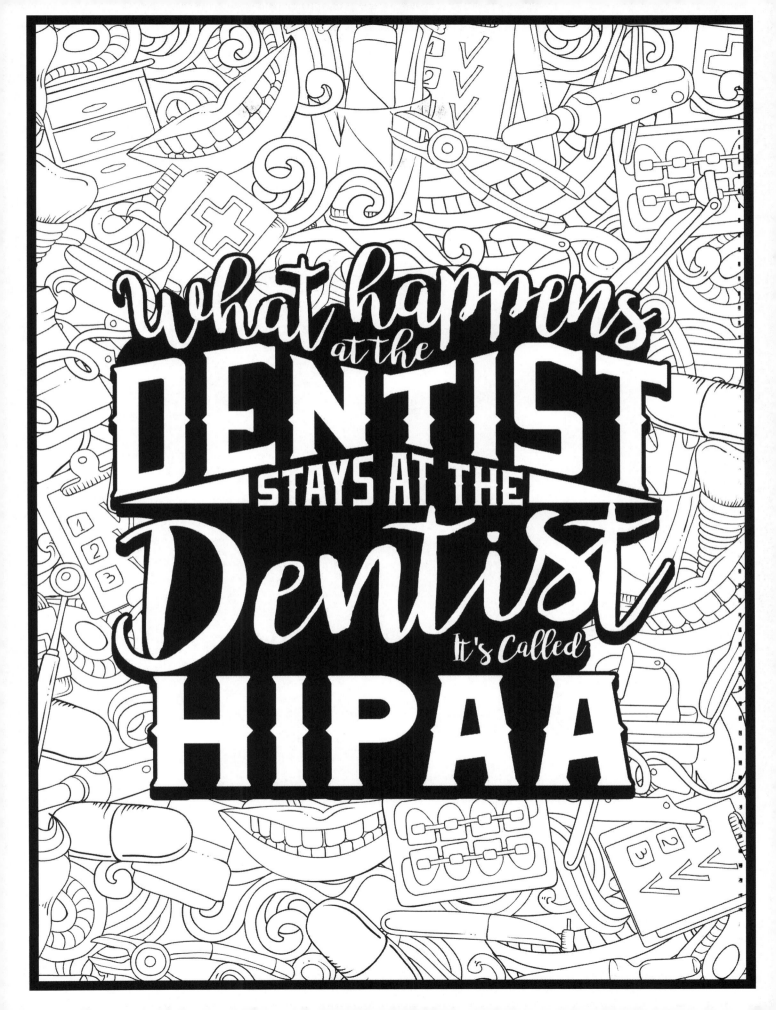

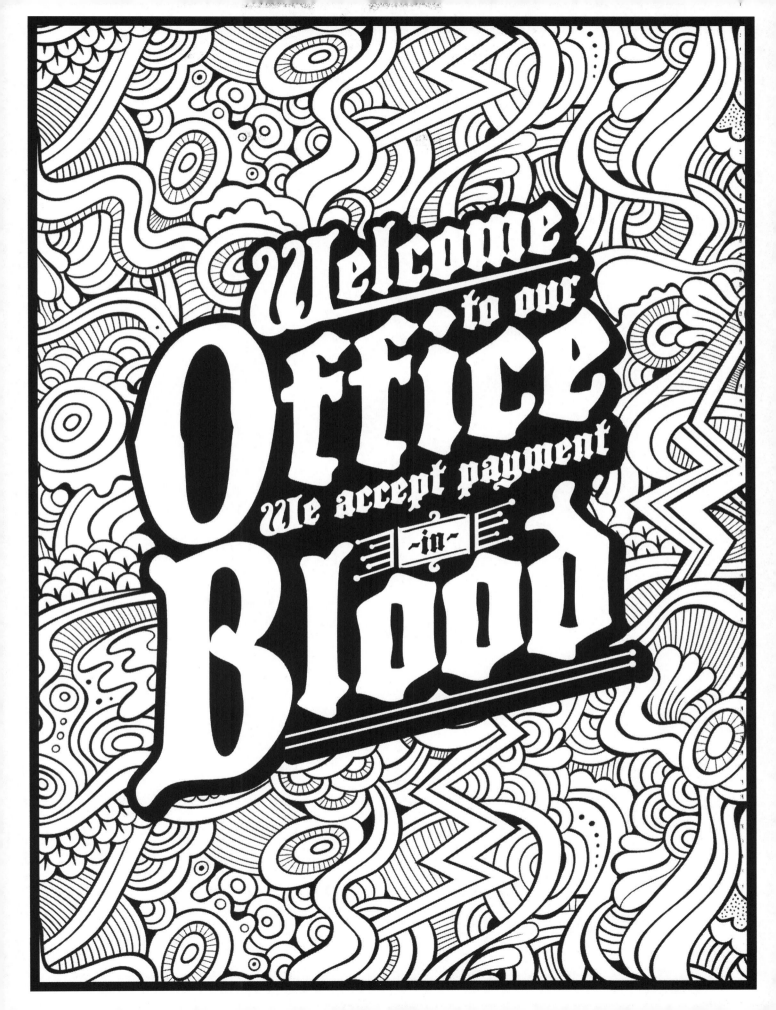

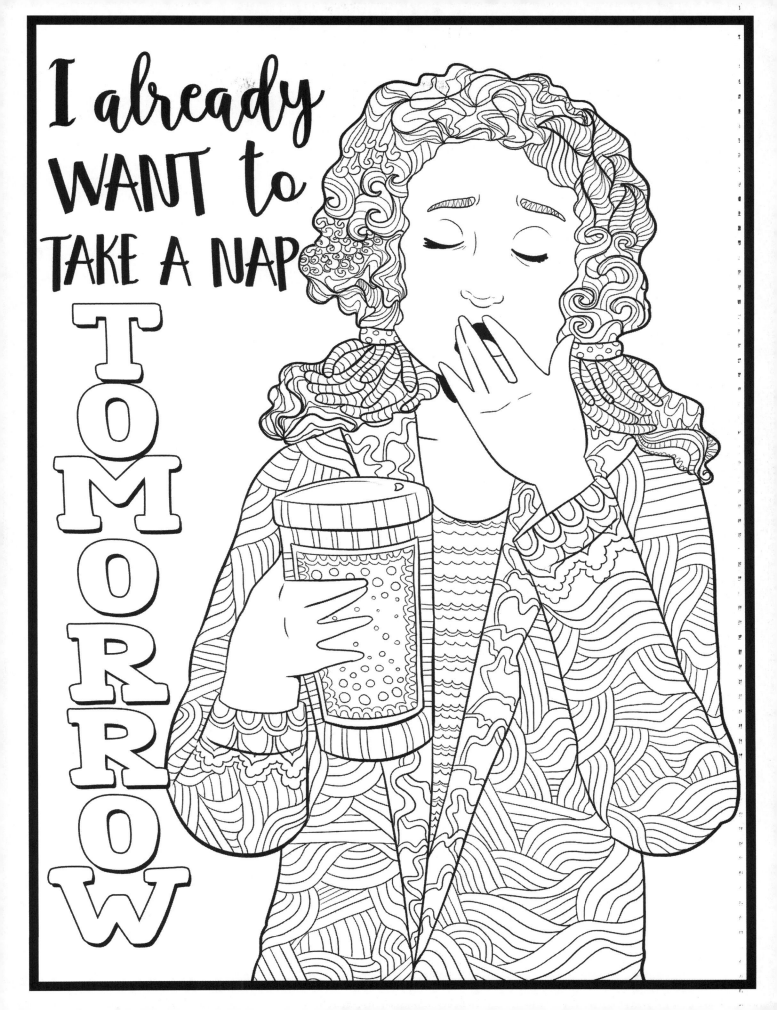

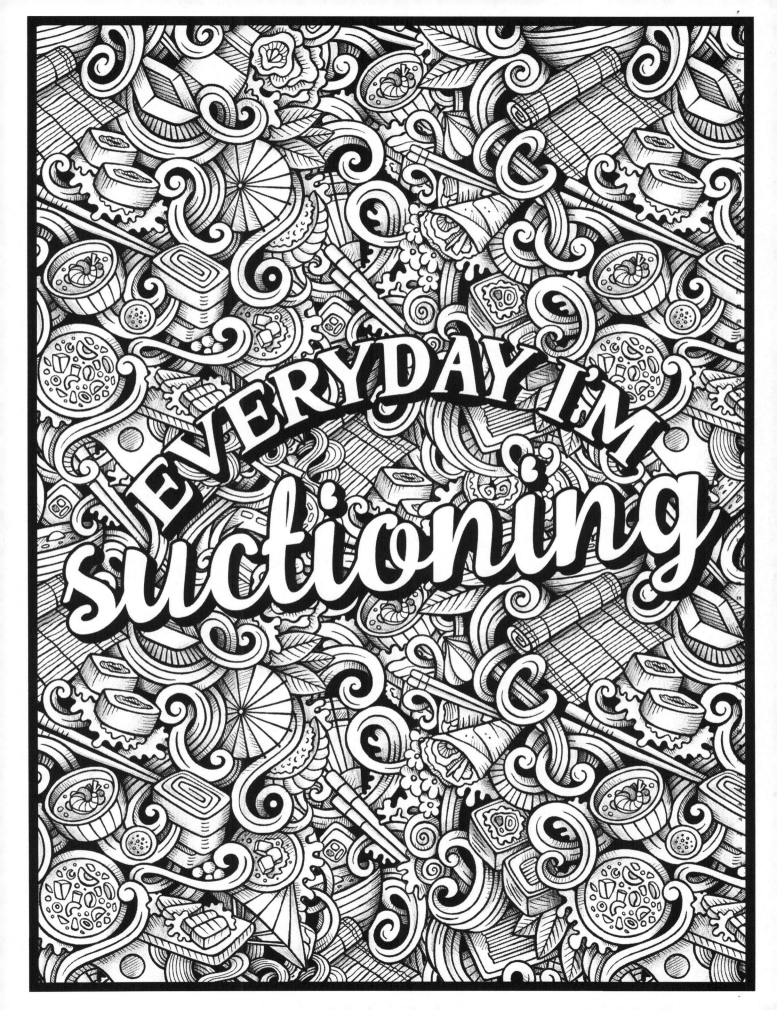

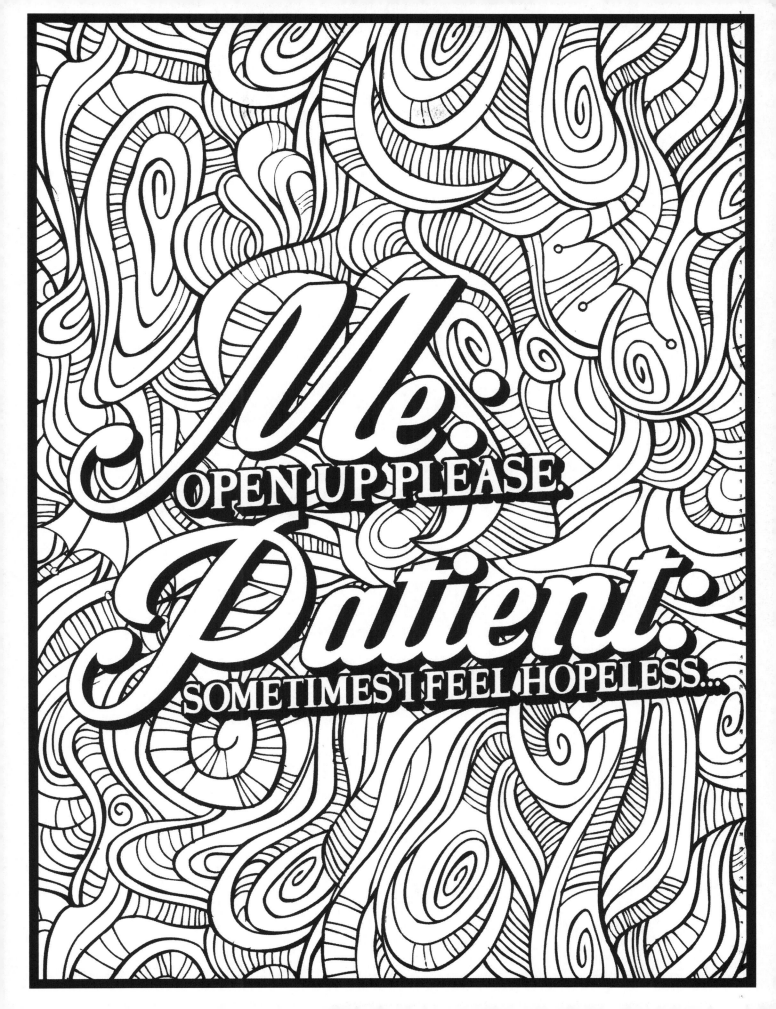

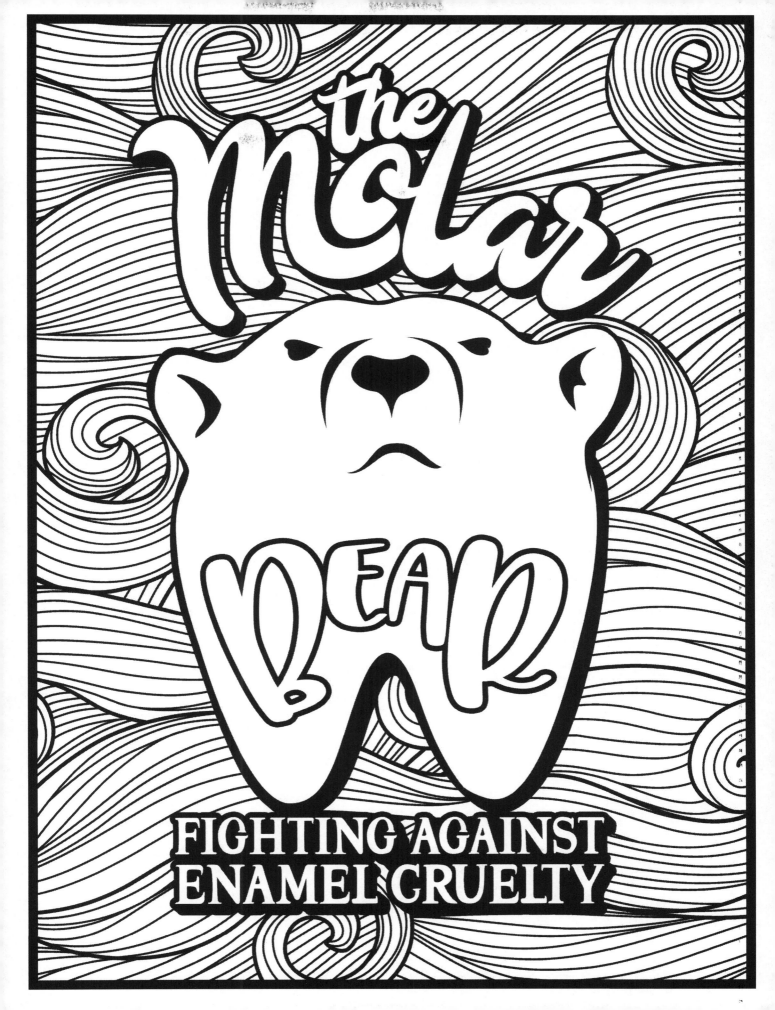

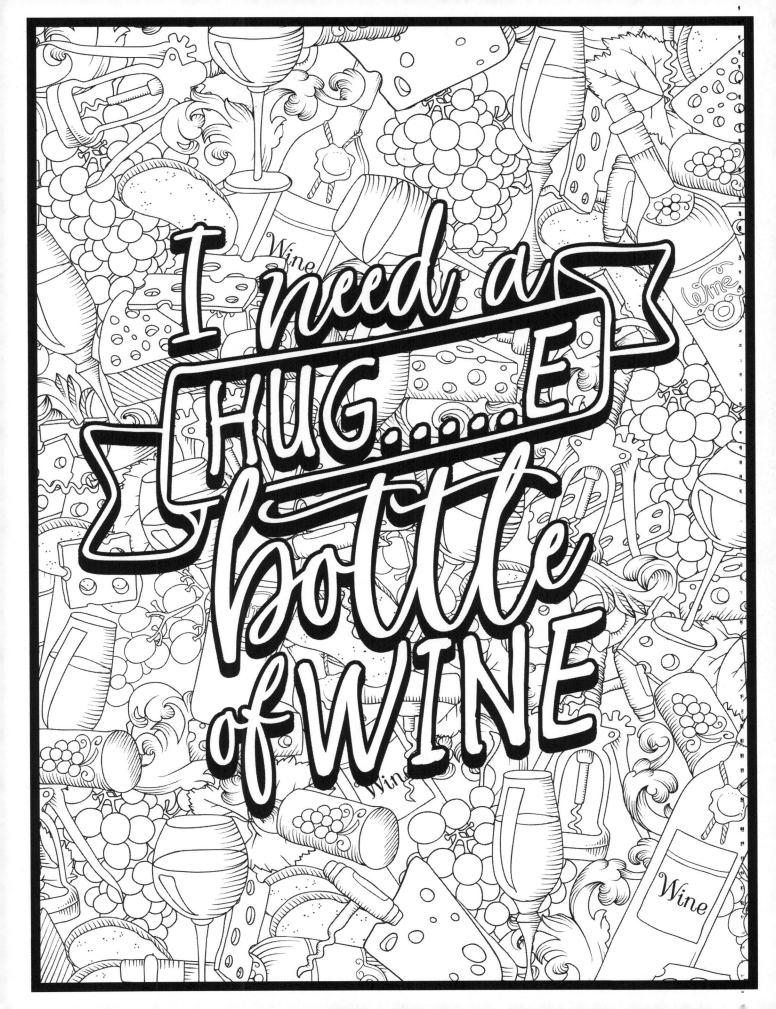

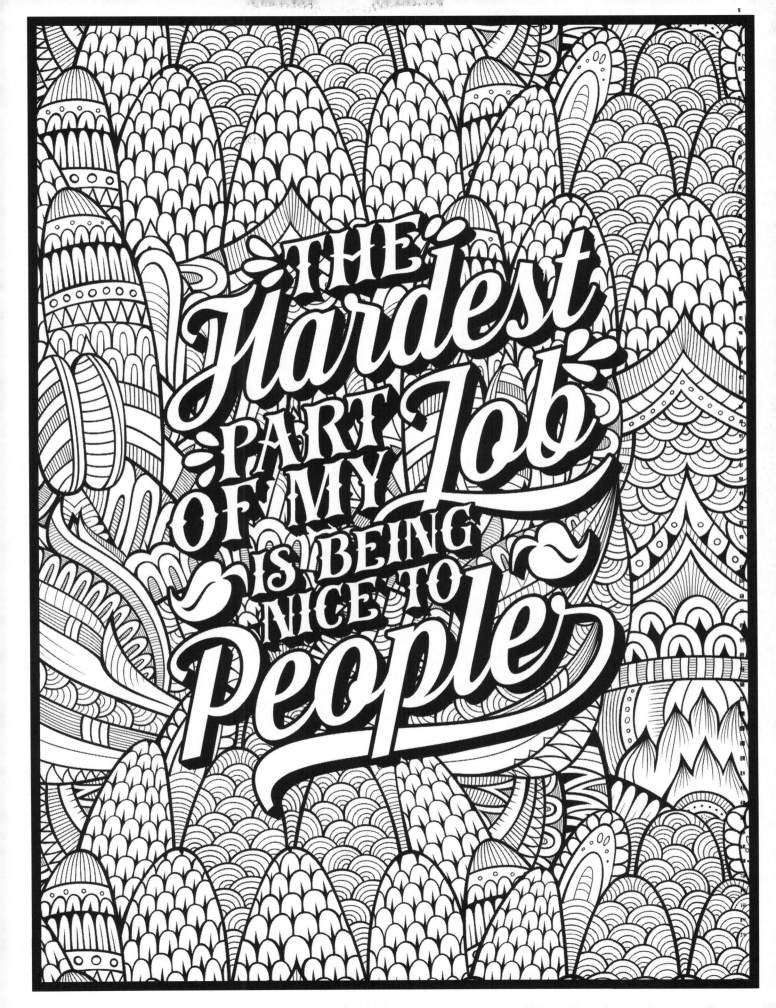

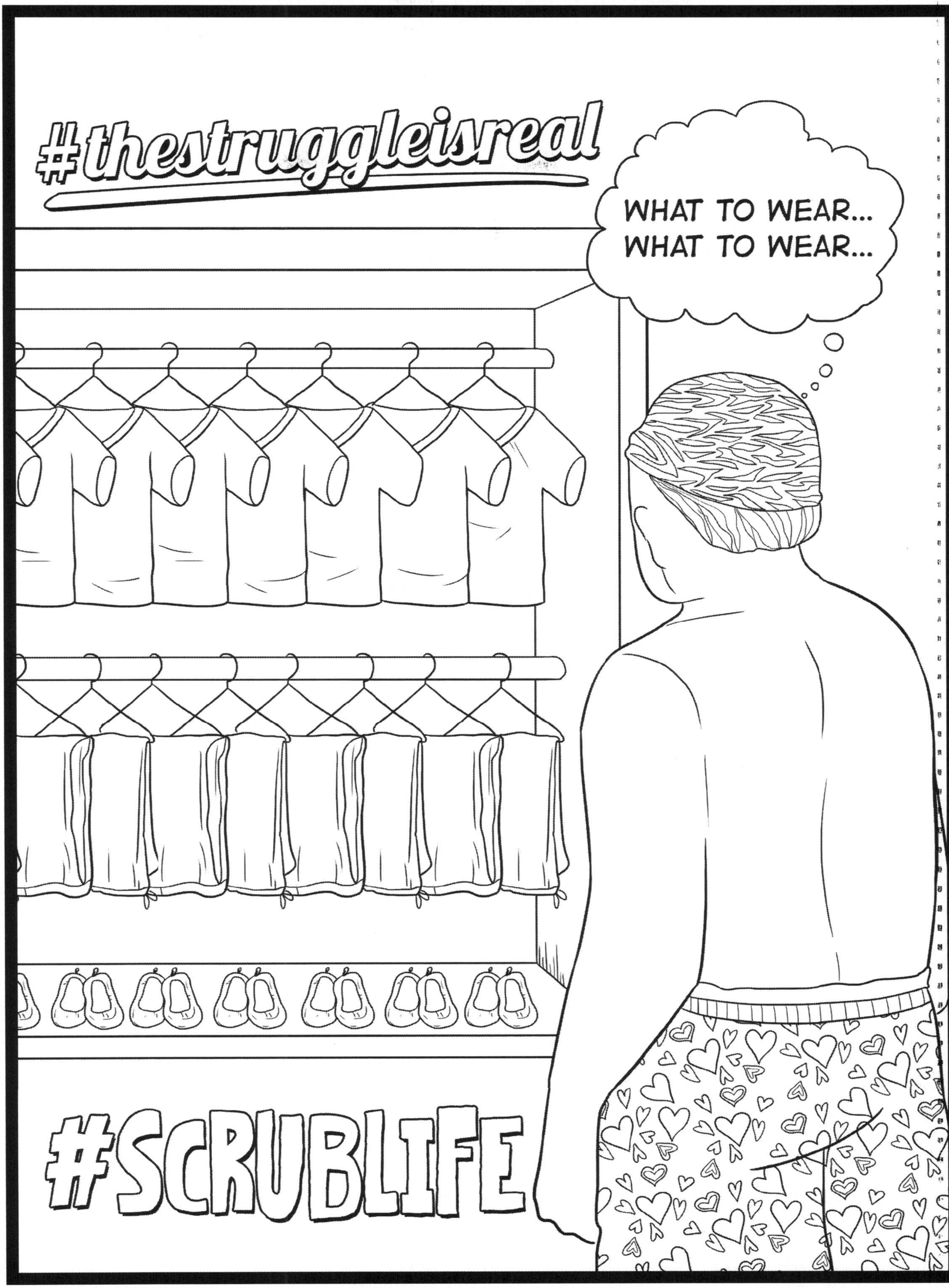
#thestruggleisreal
WHAT TO WEAR...
WHAT TO WEAR...
#SCRUBLIFE

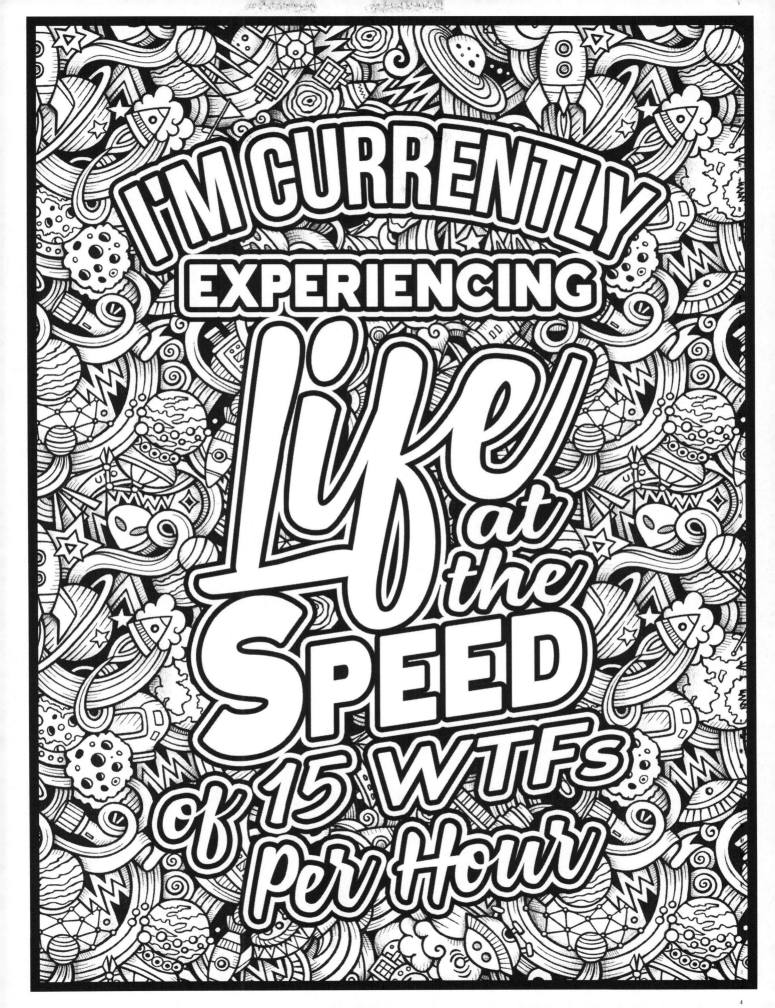

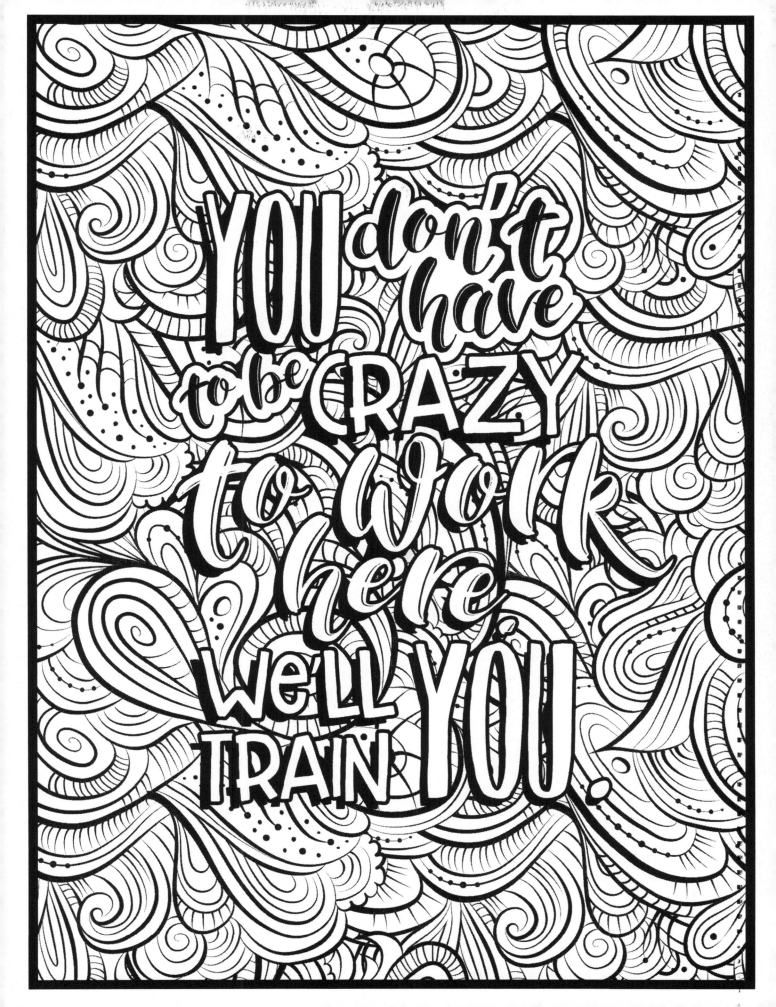

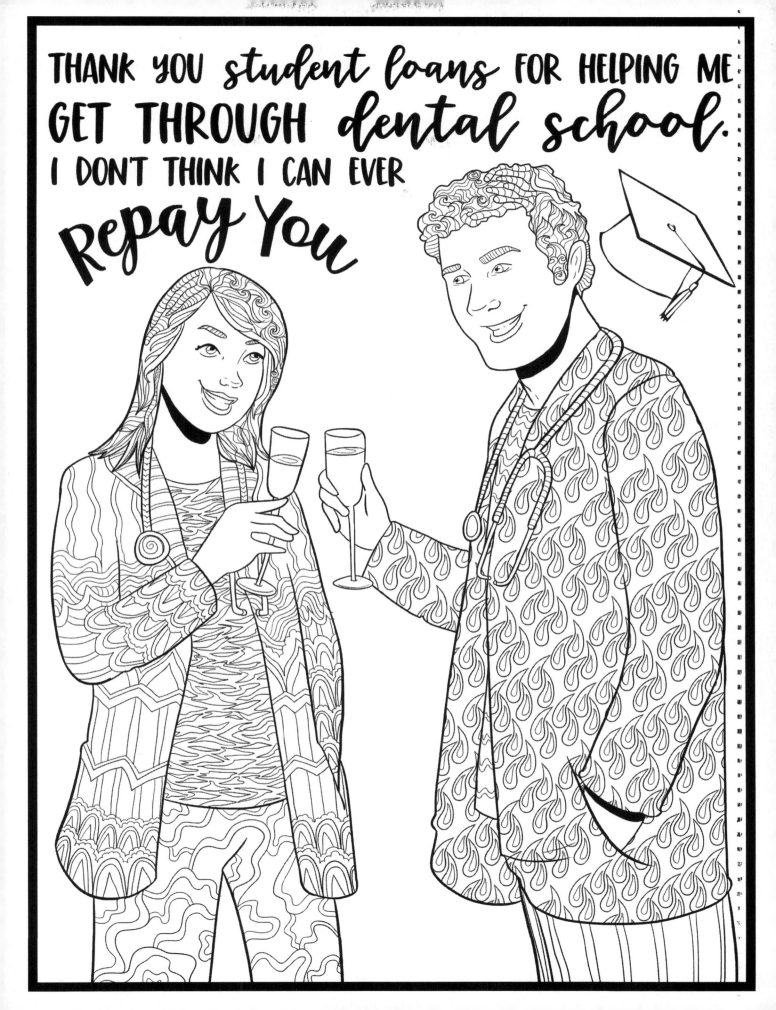

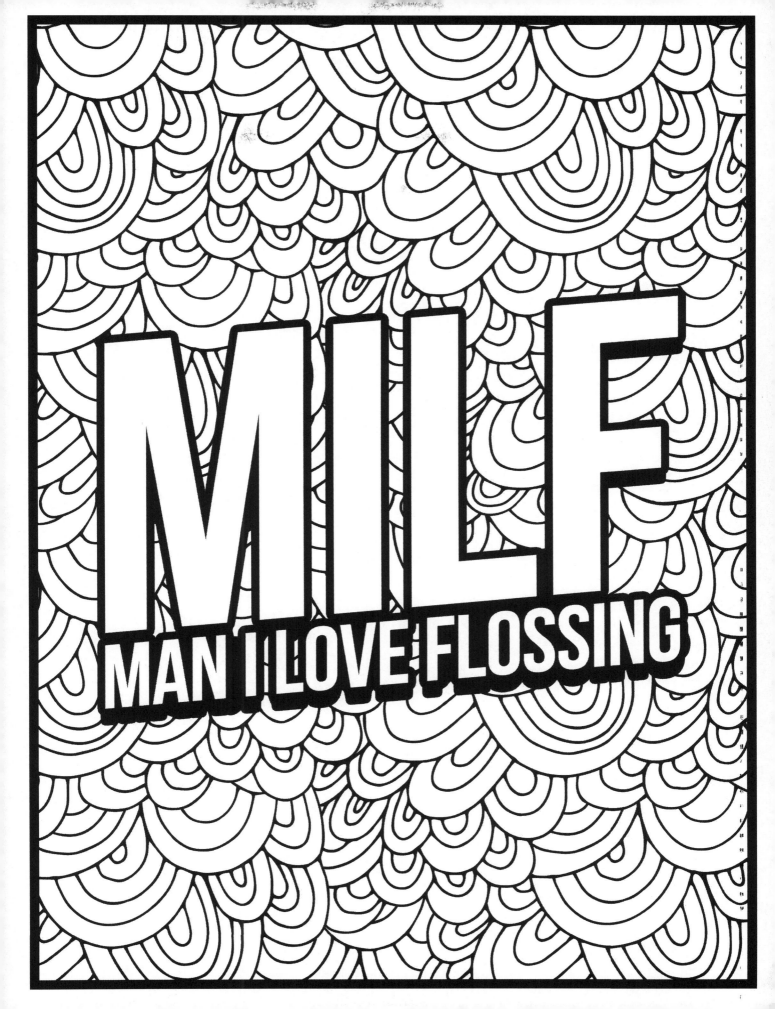

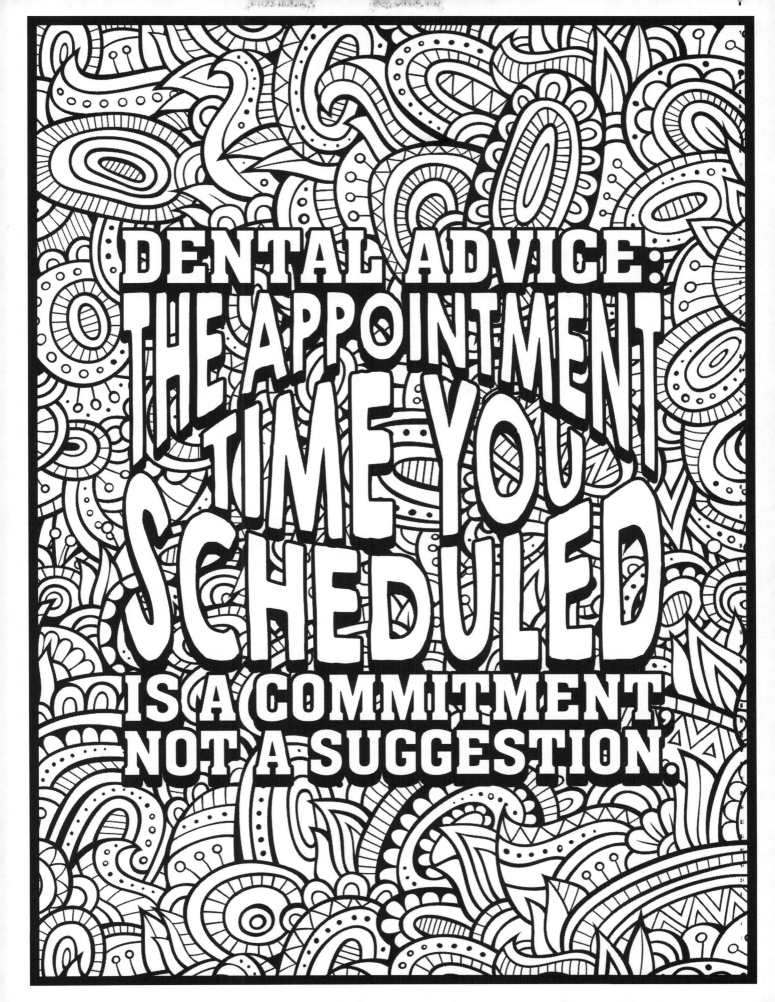

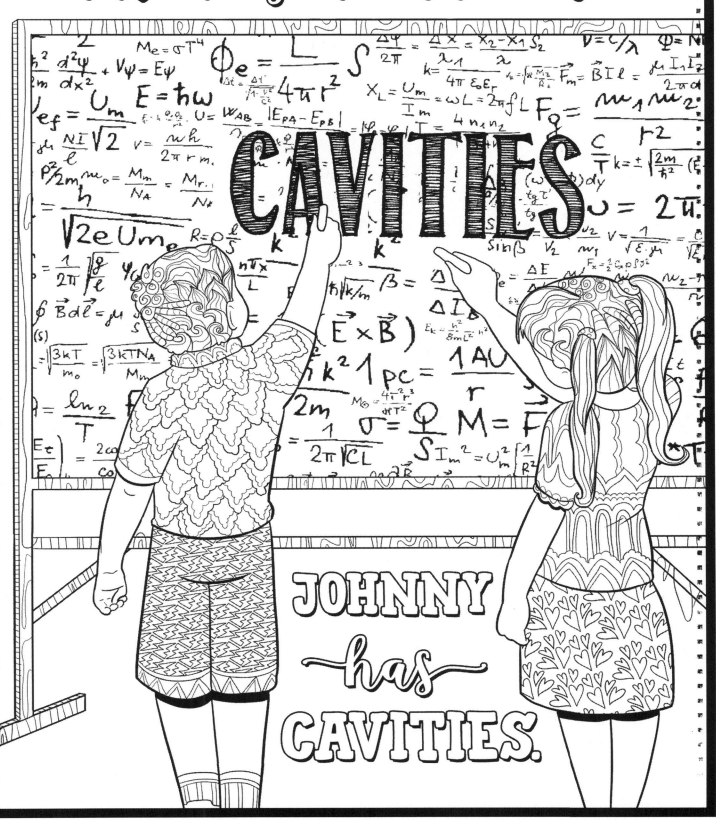

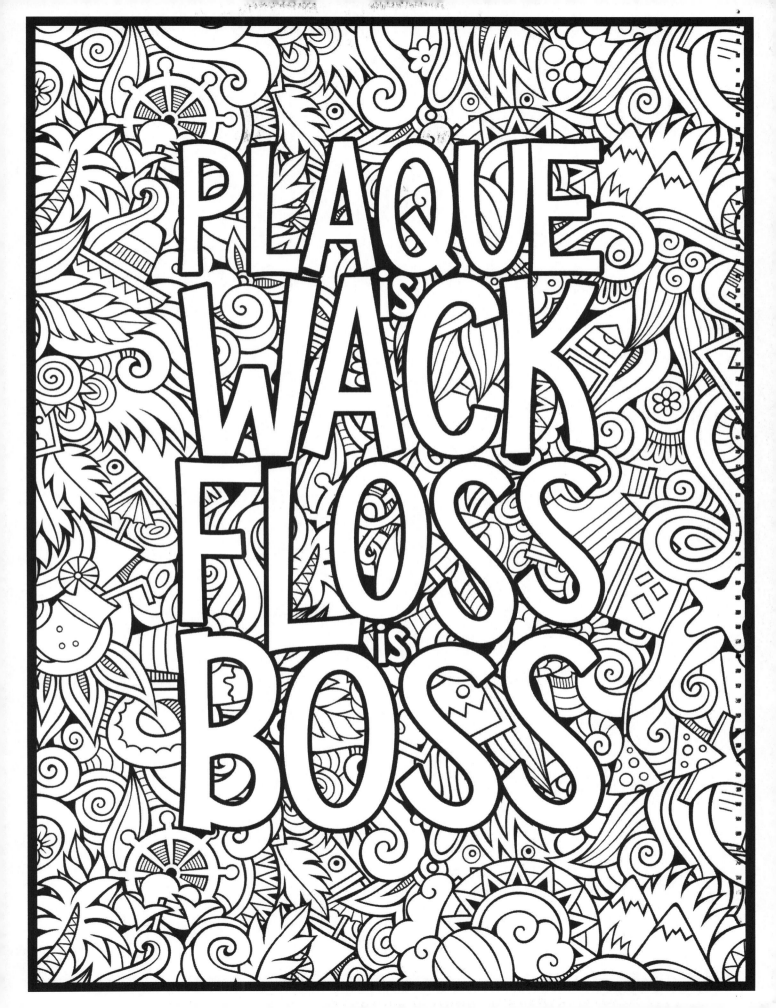

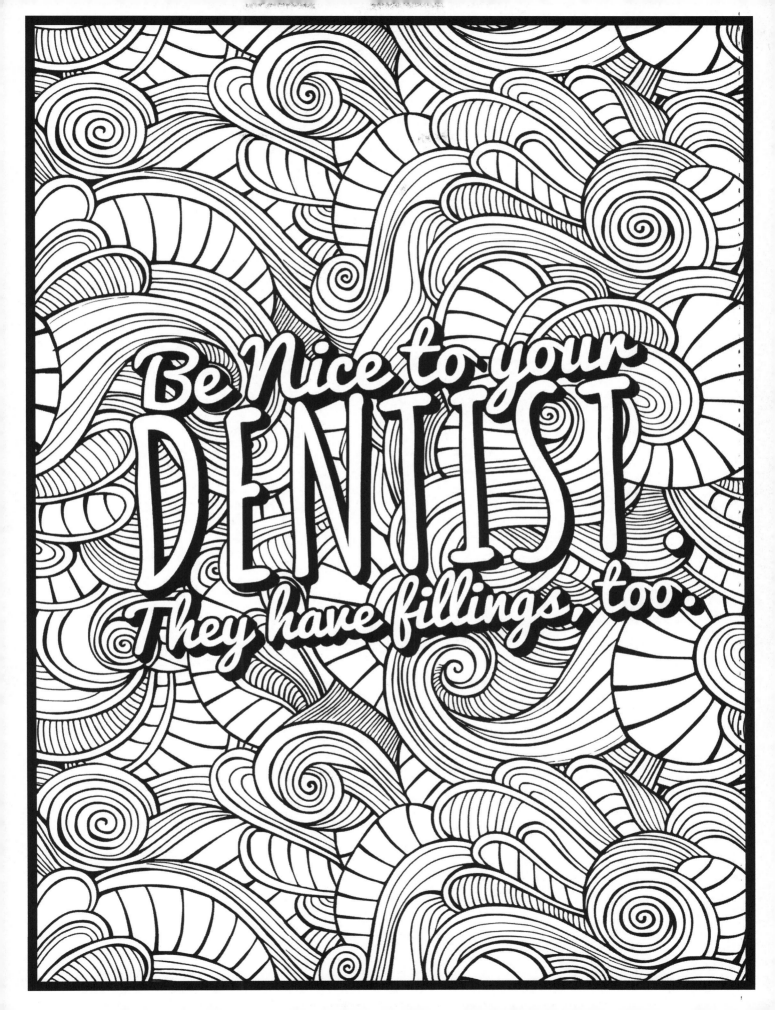

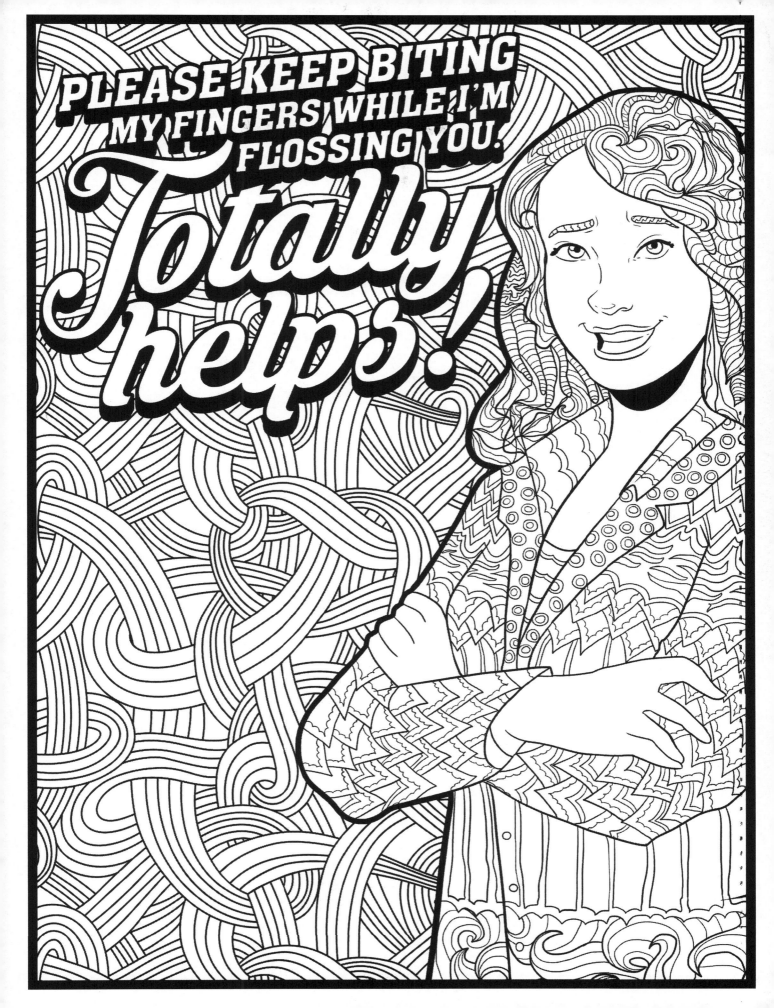

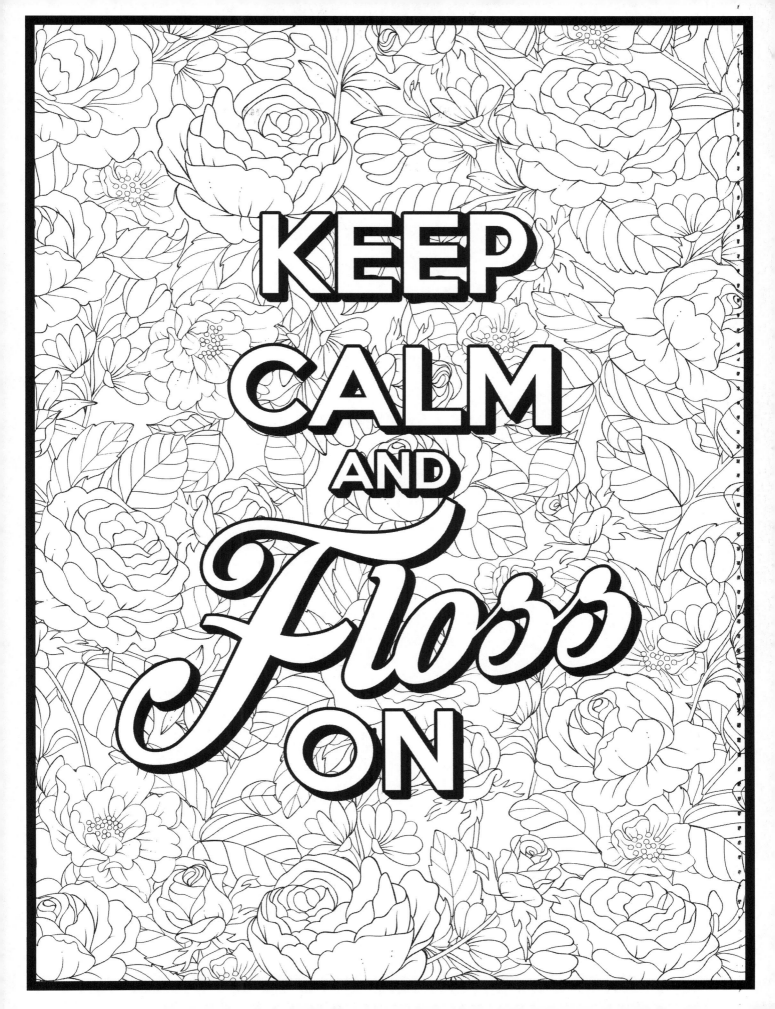

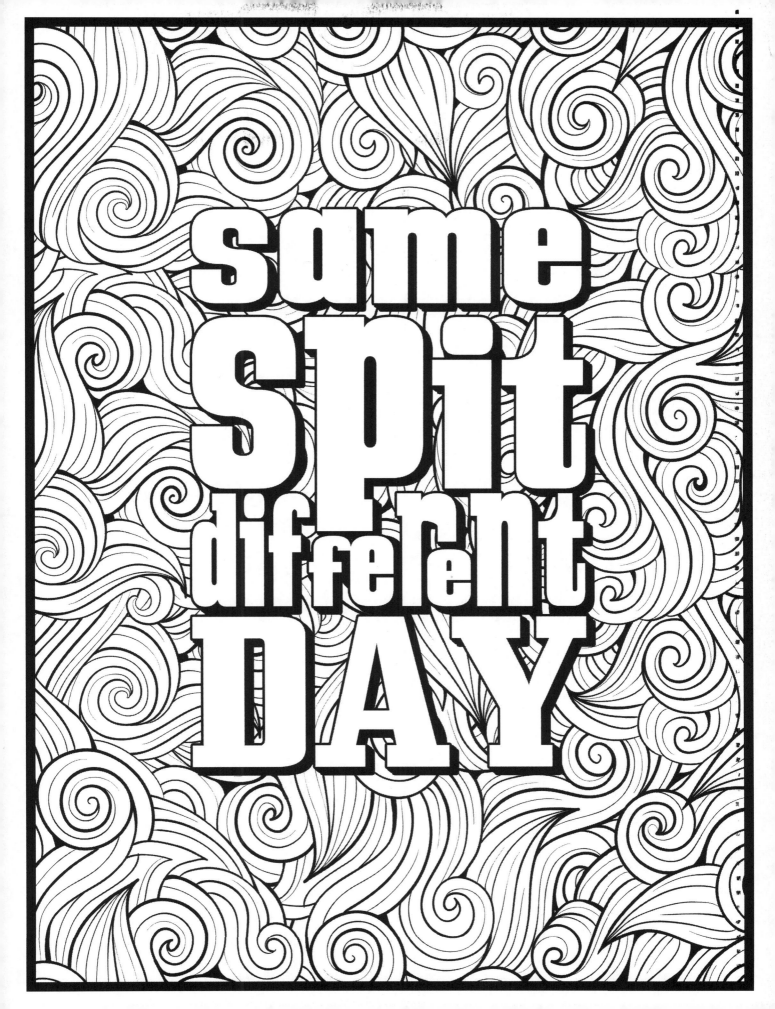

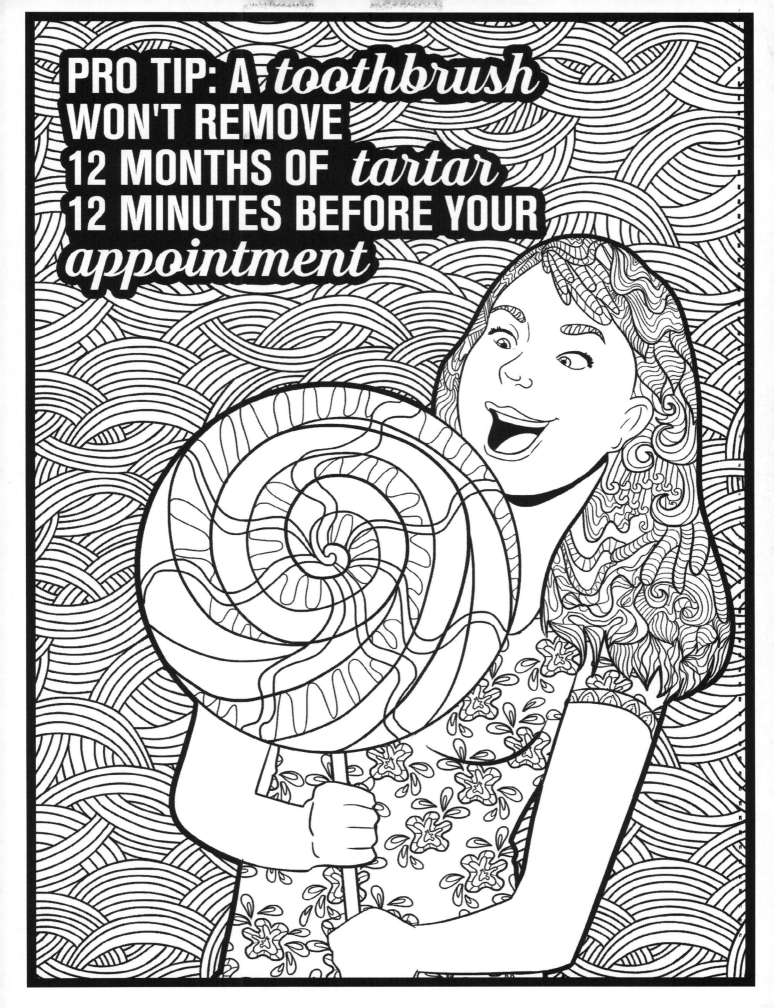

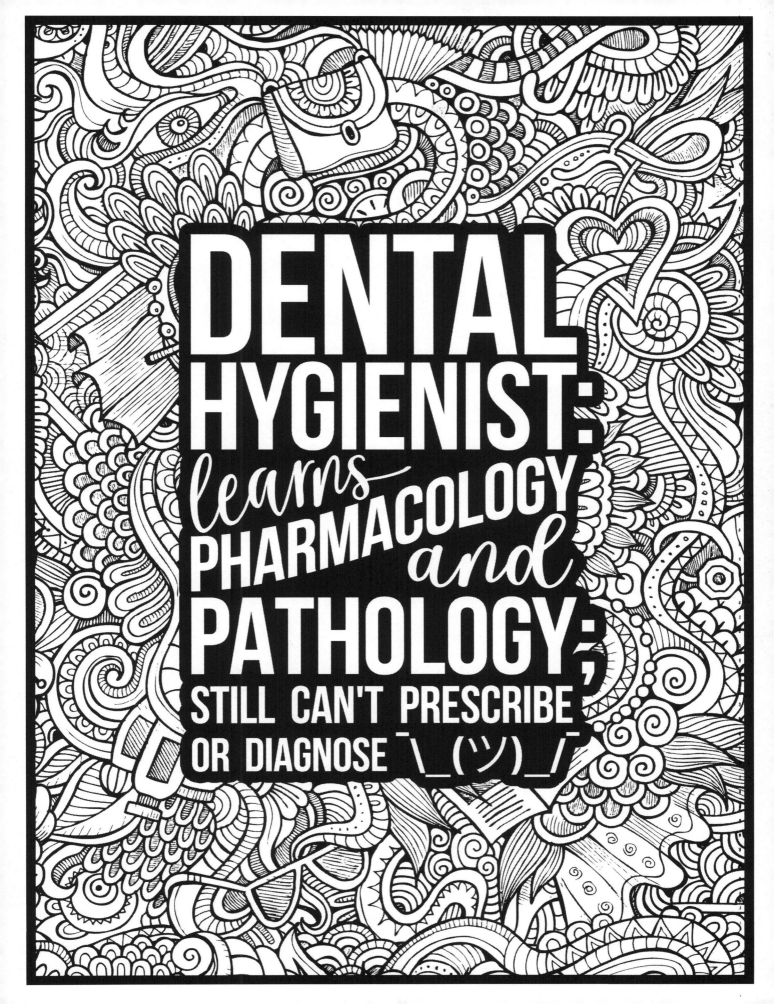

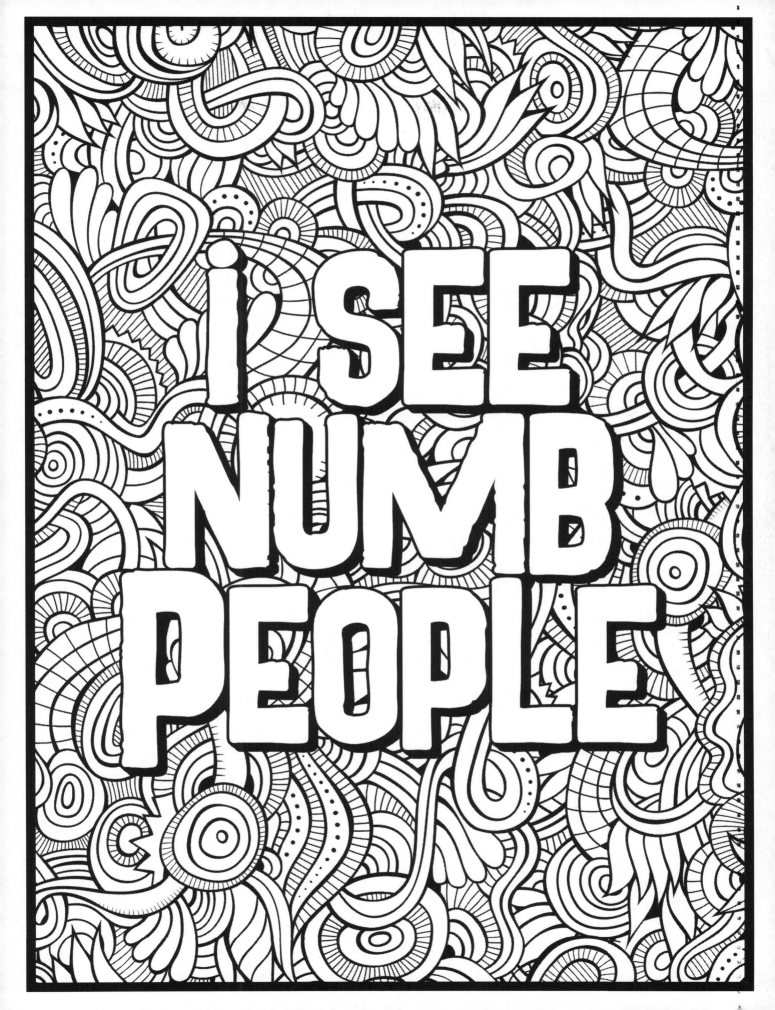

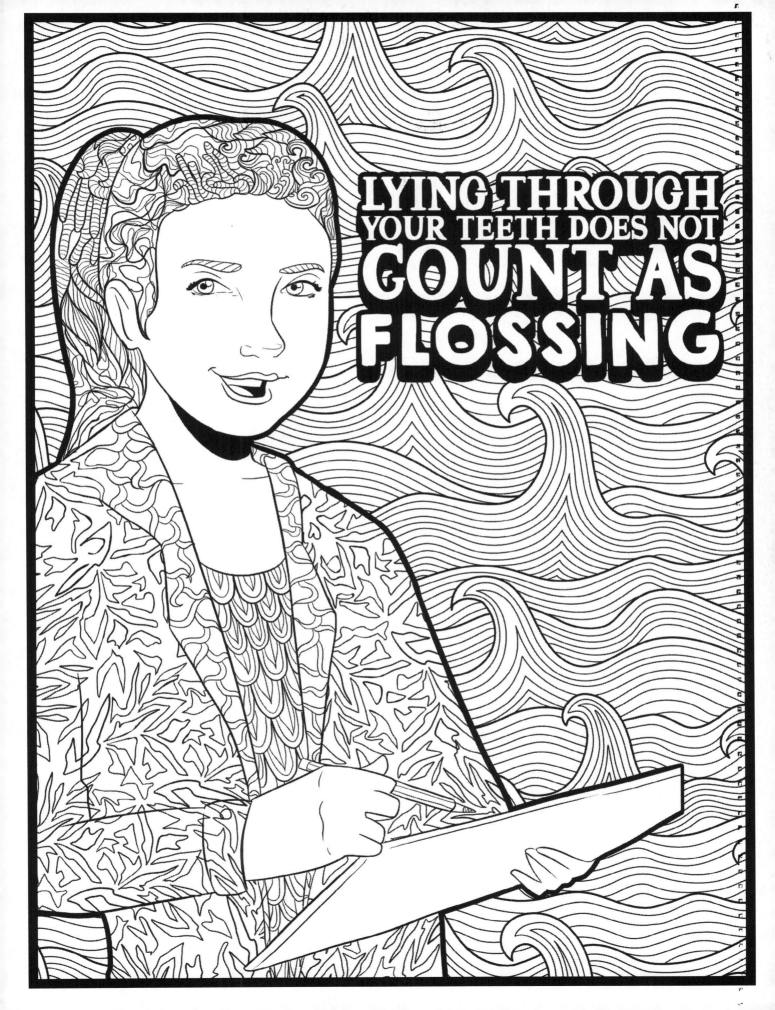

LIVIN' THE SCRUB LIFE

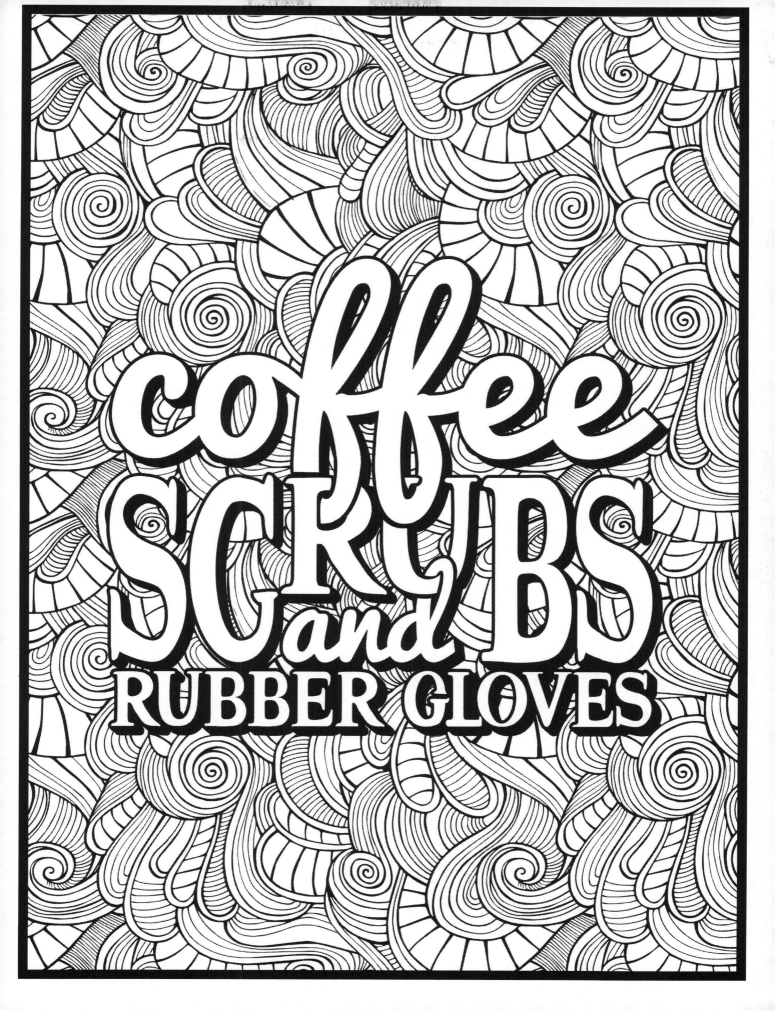

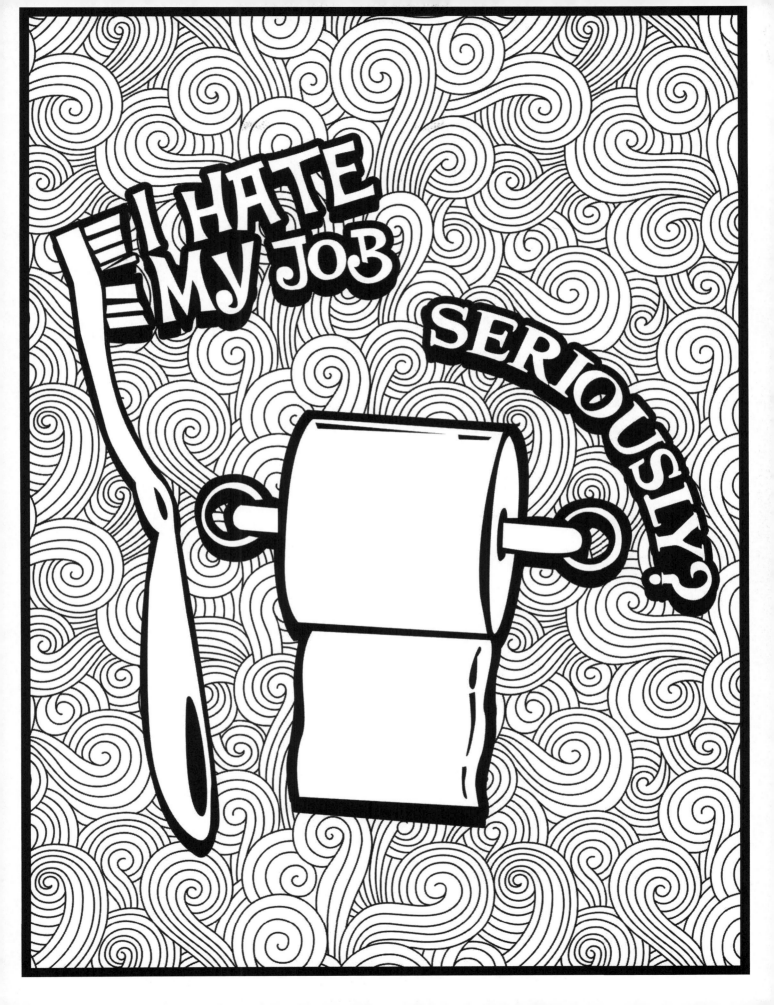

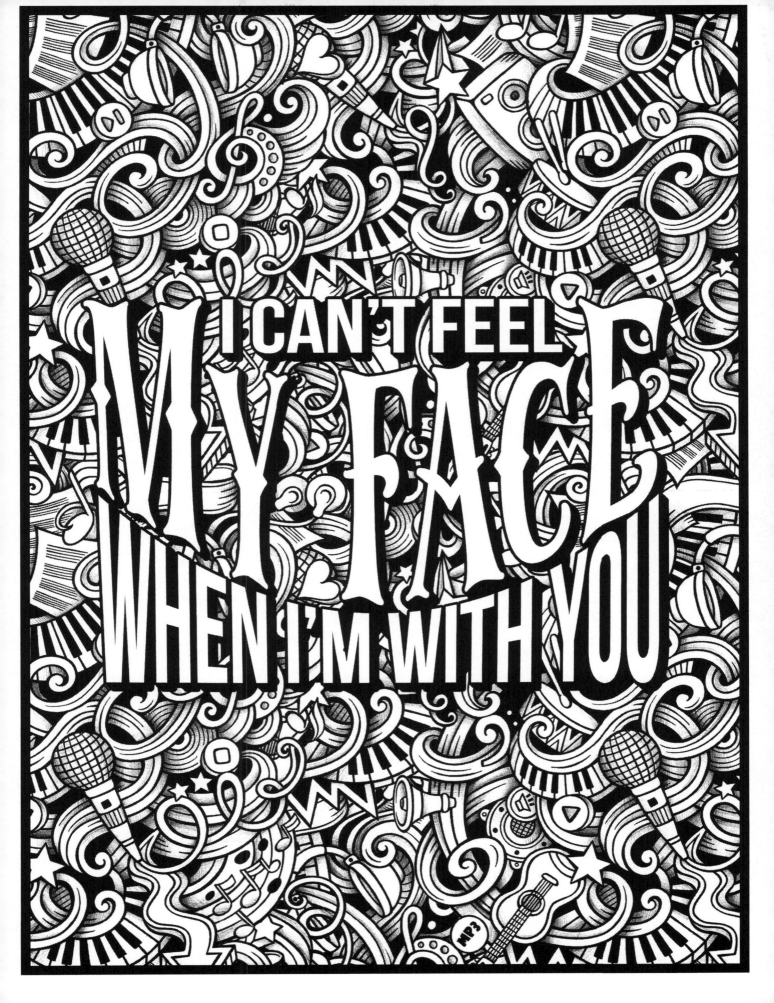

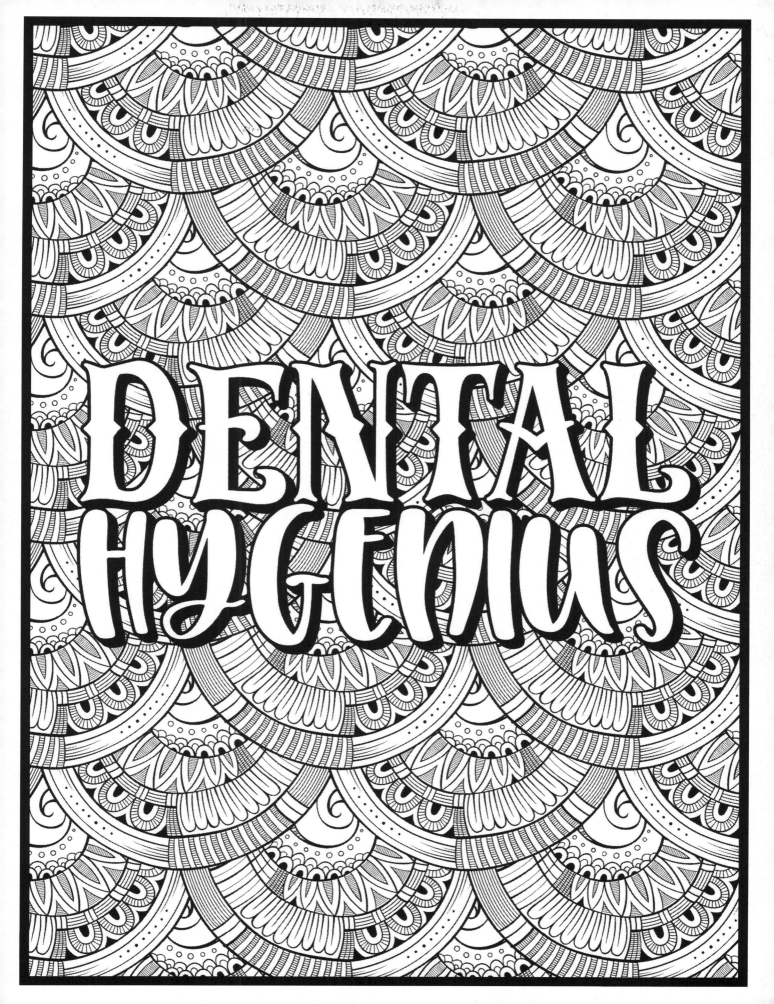

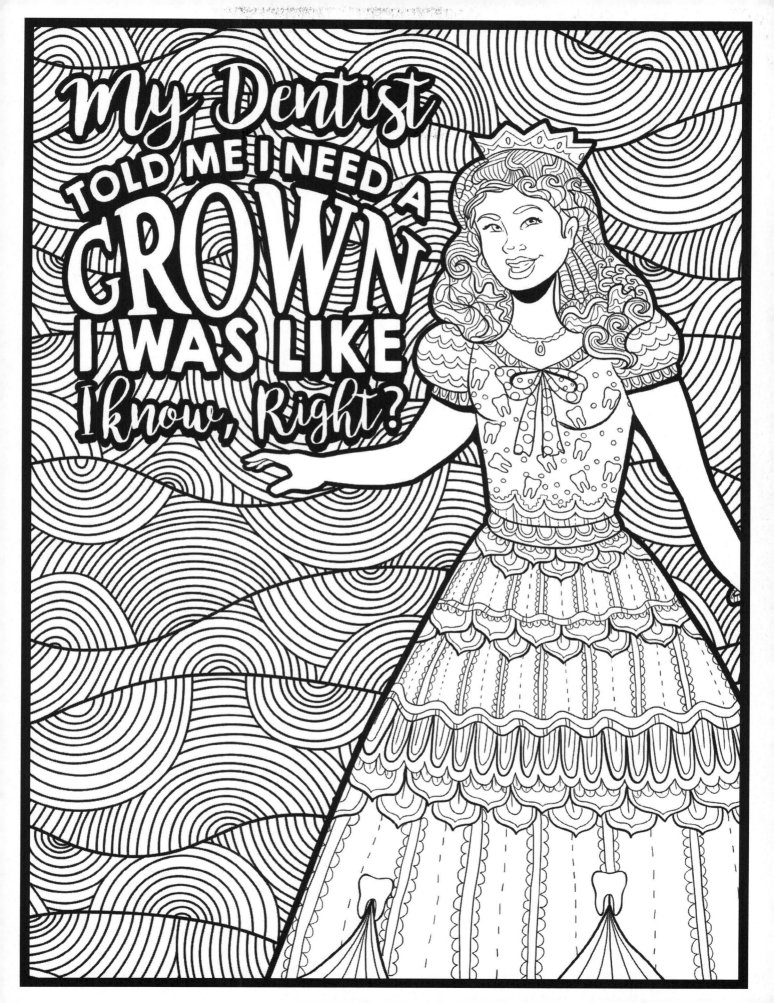

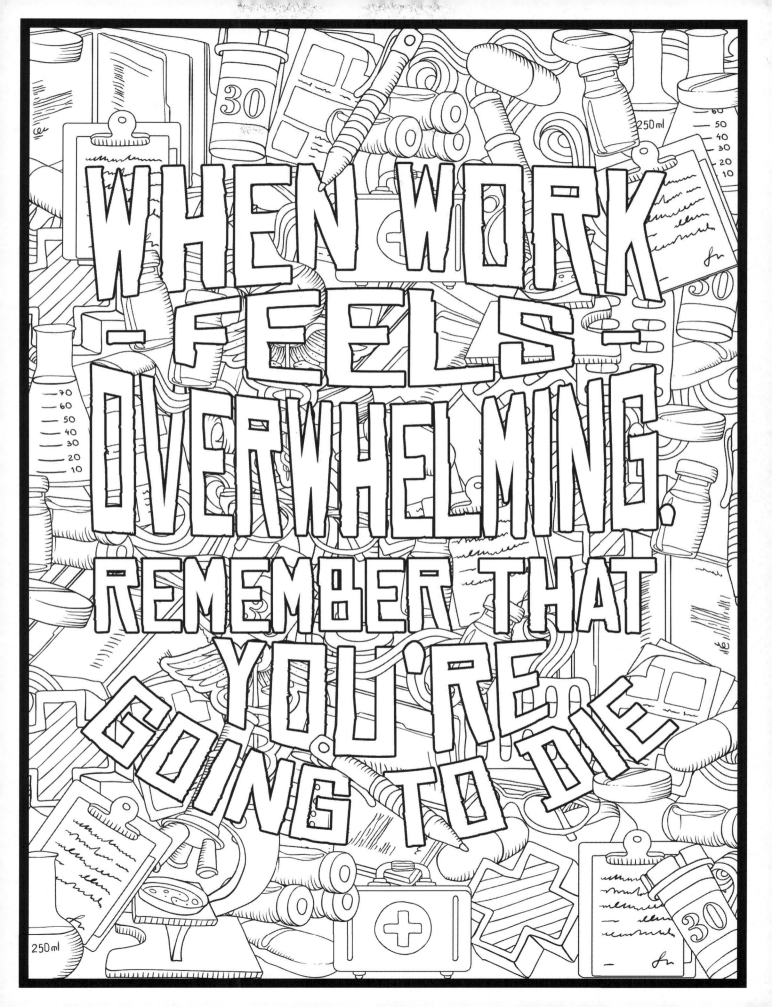

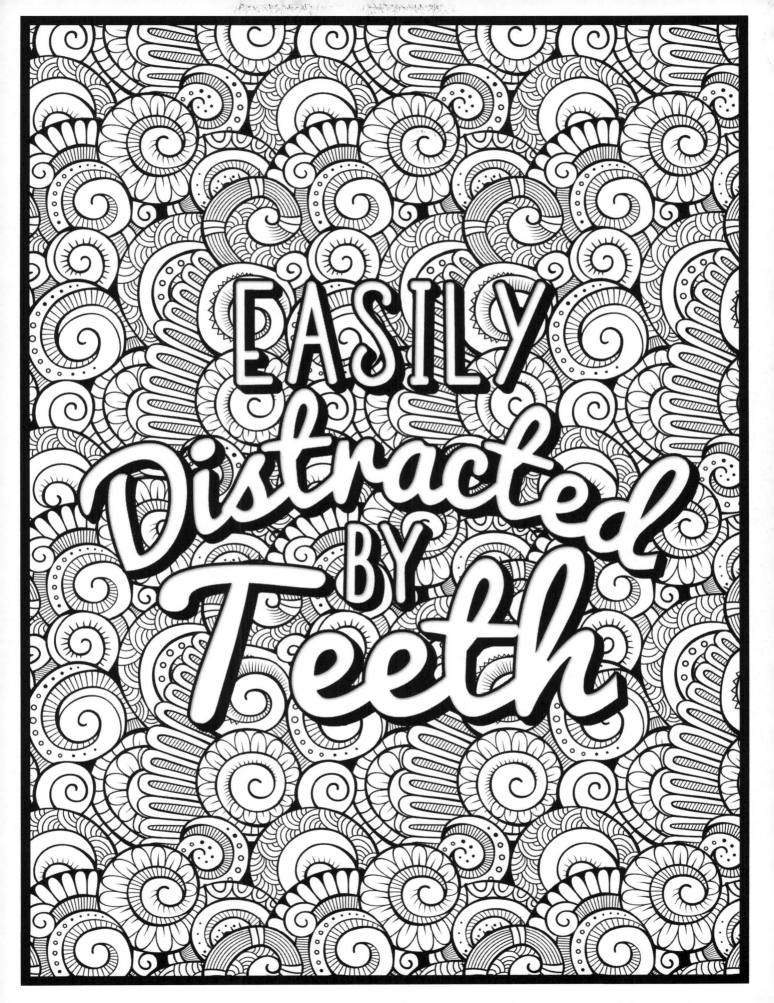

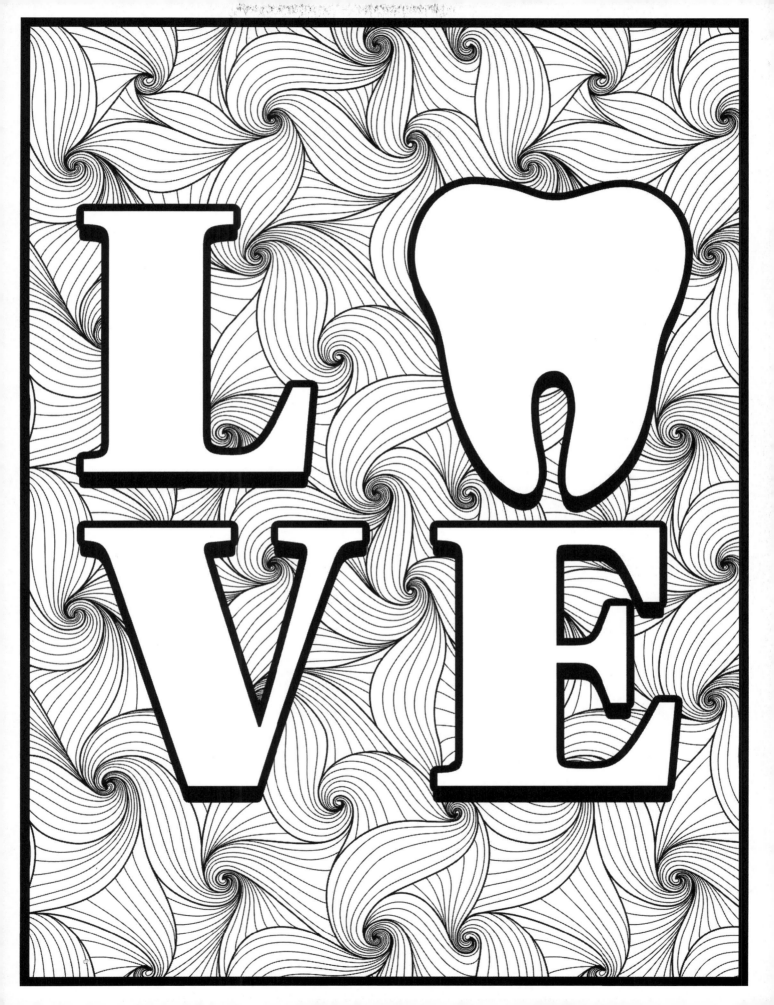

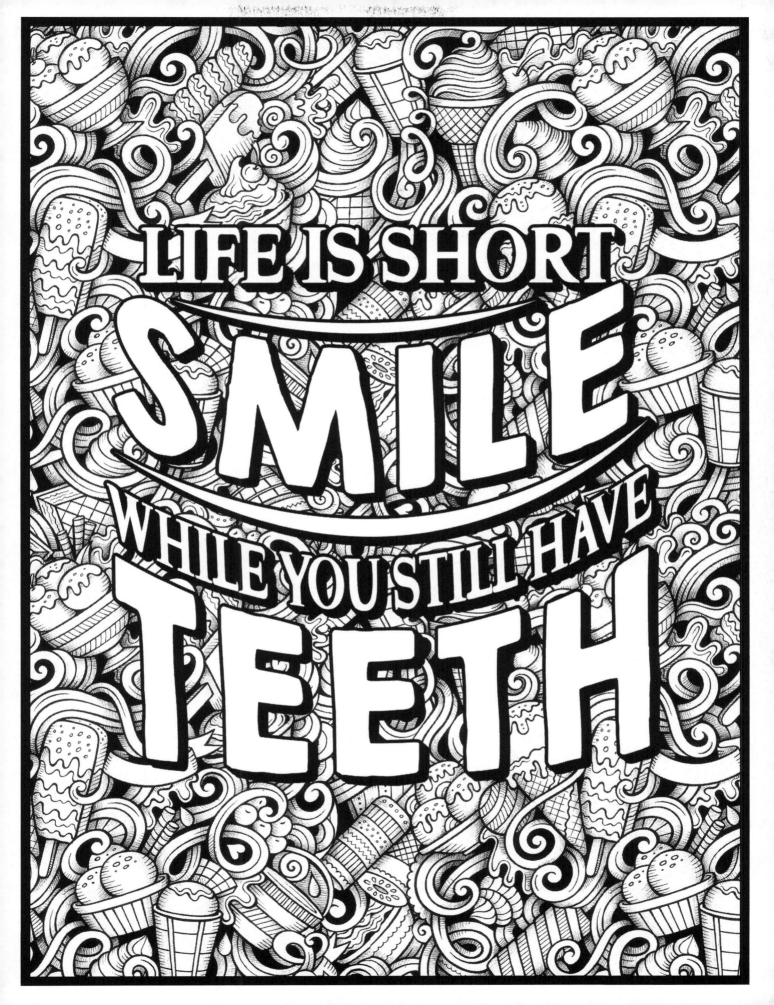

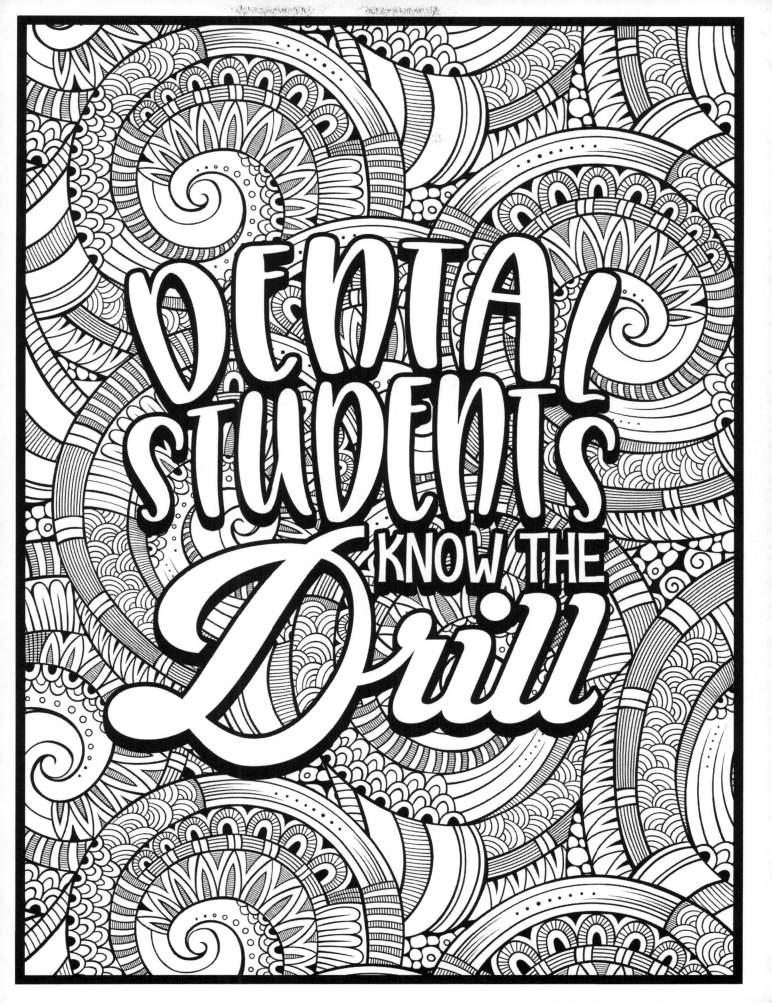

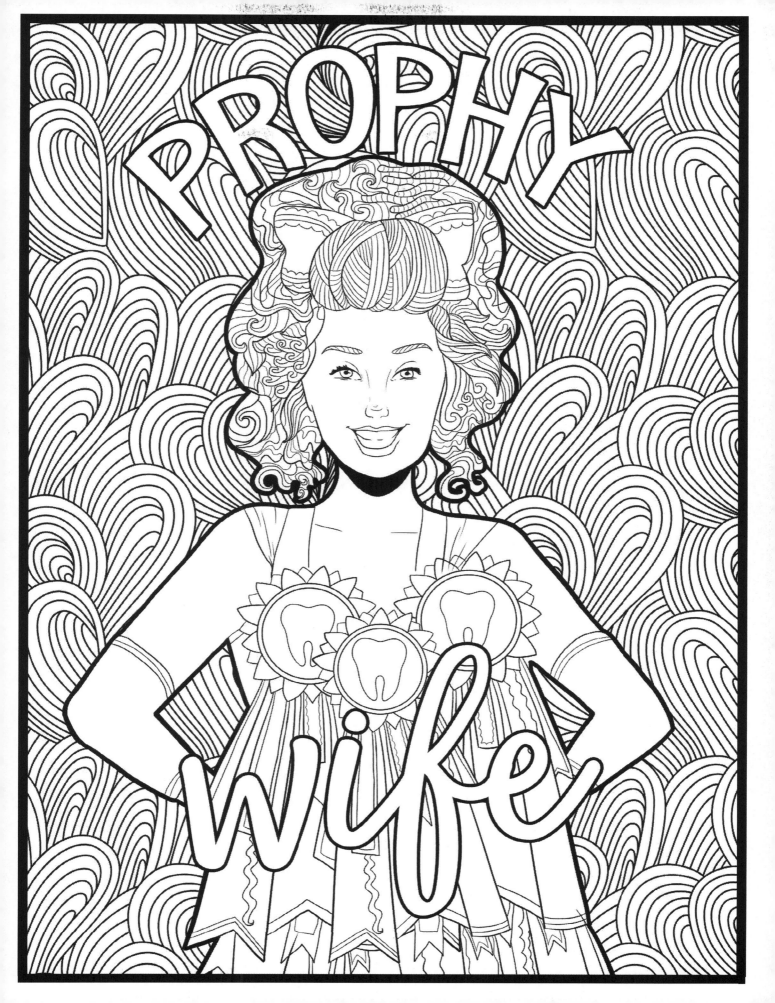

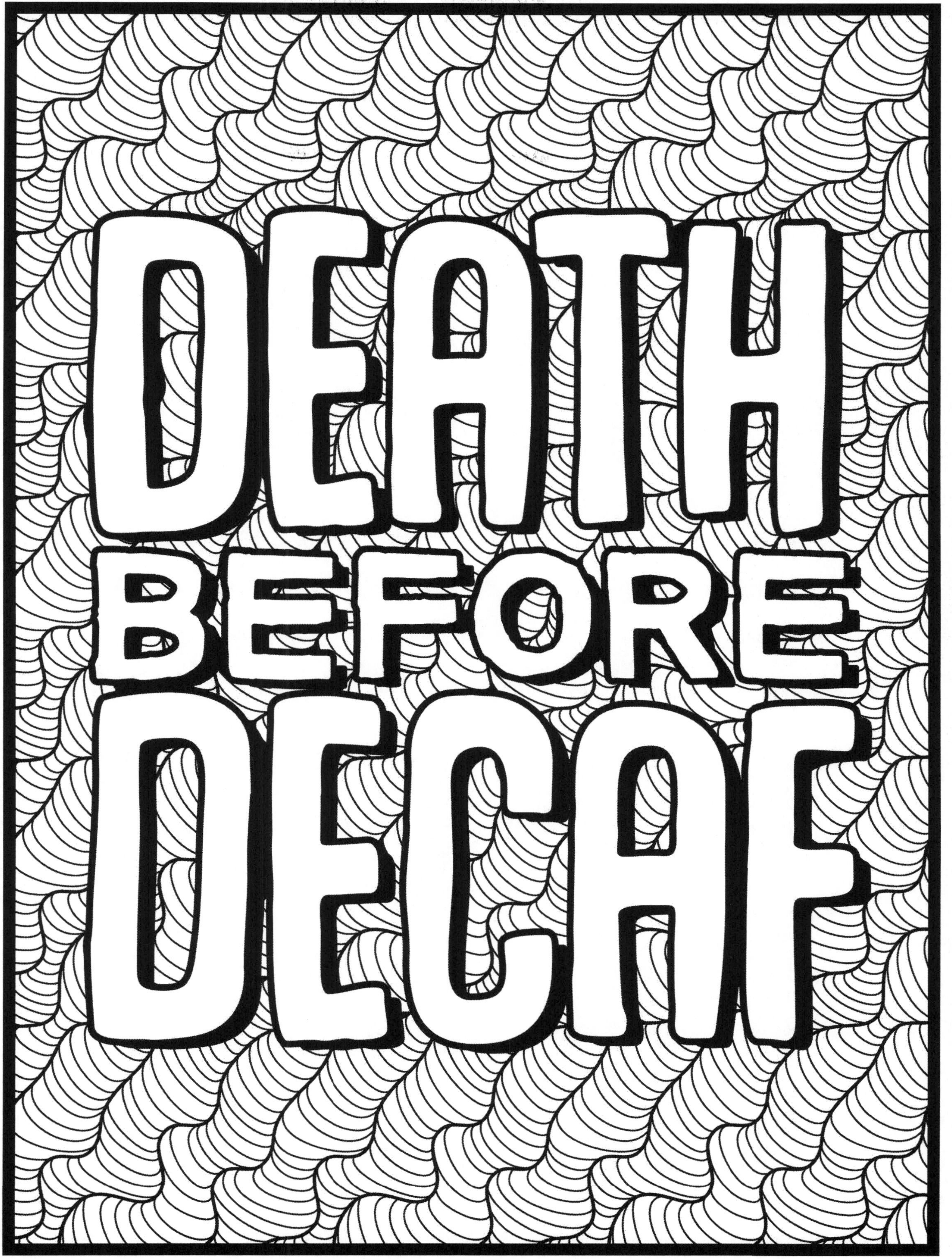
DEATH
BEFORE
DECAF

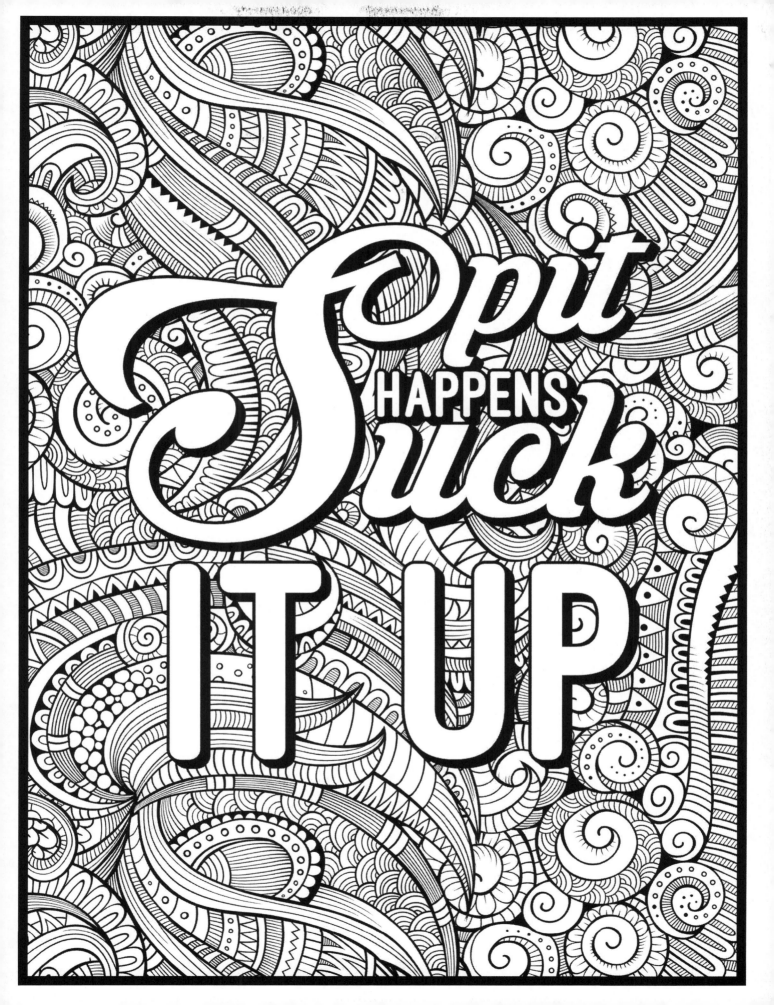

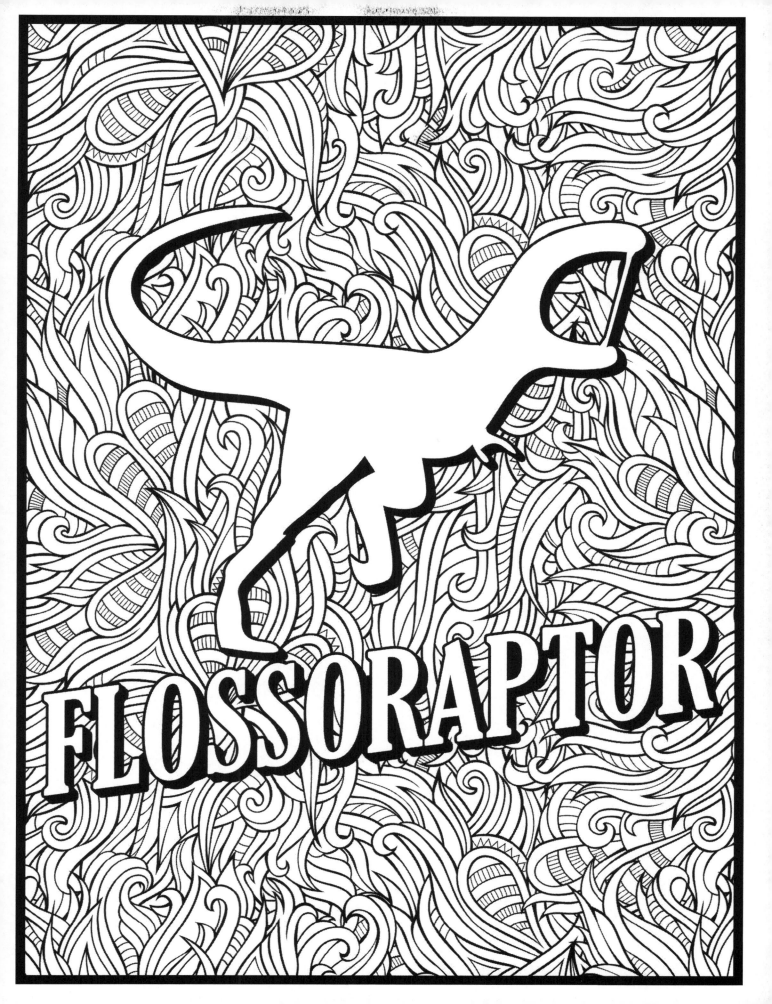

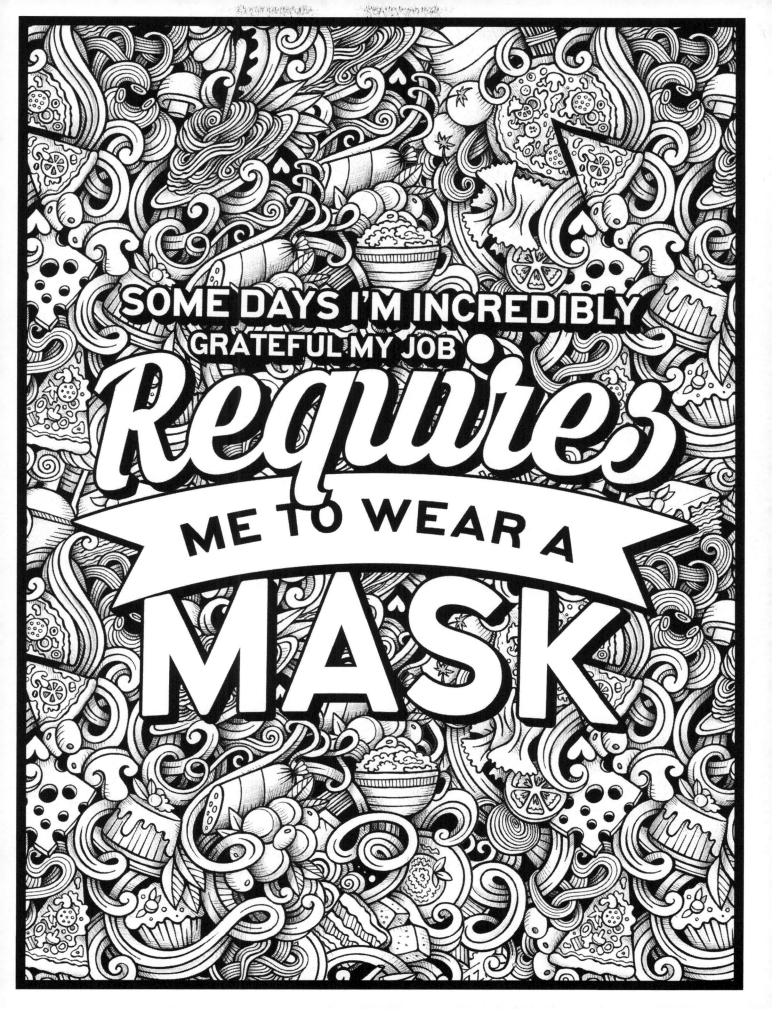

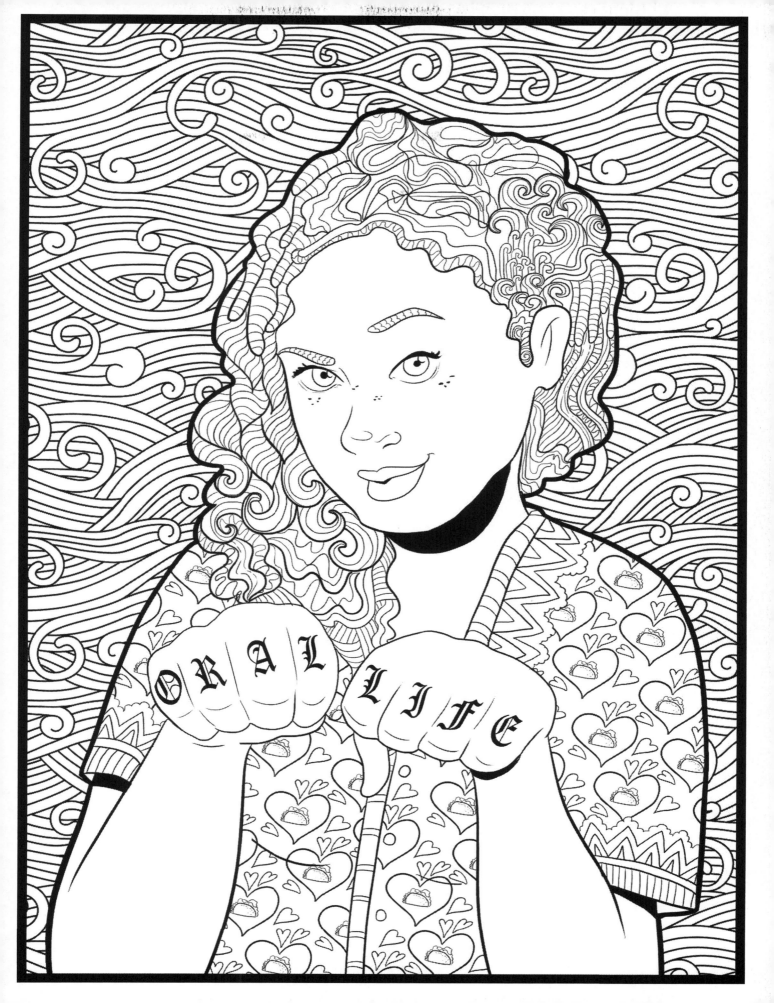

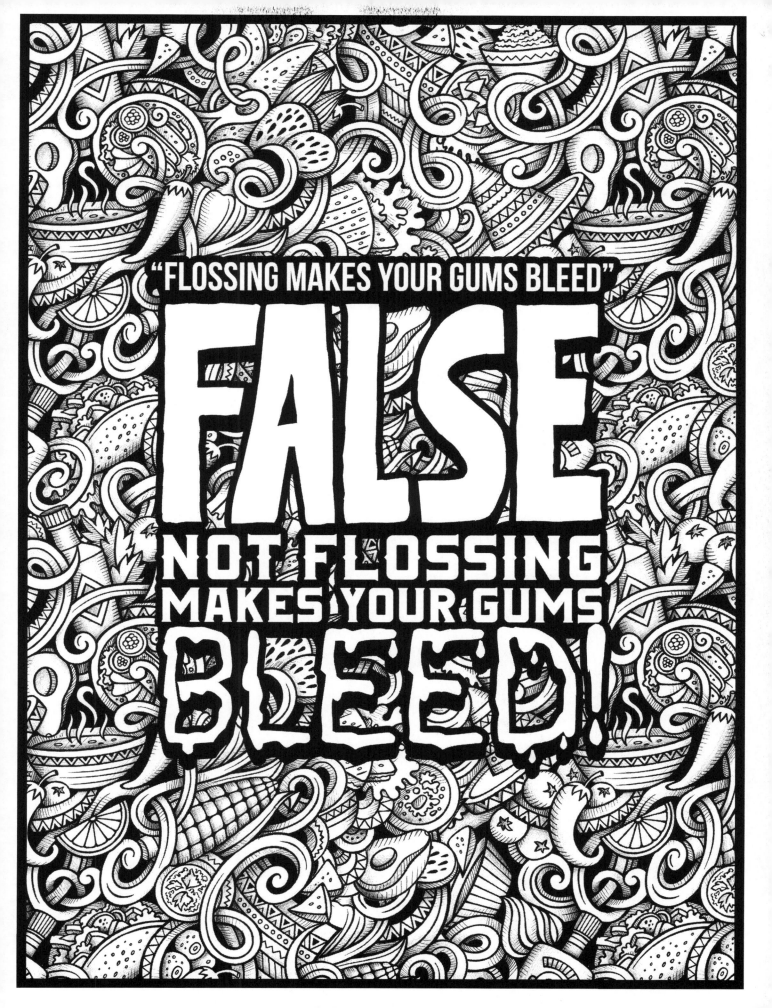

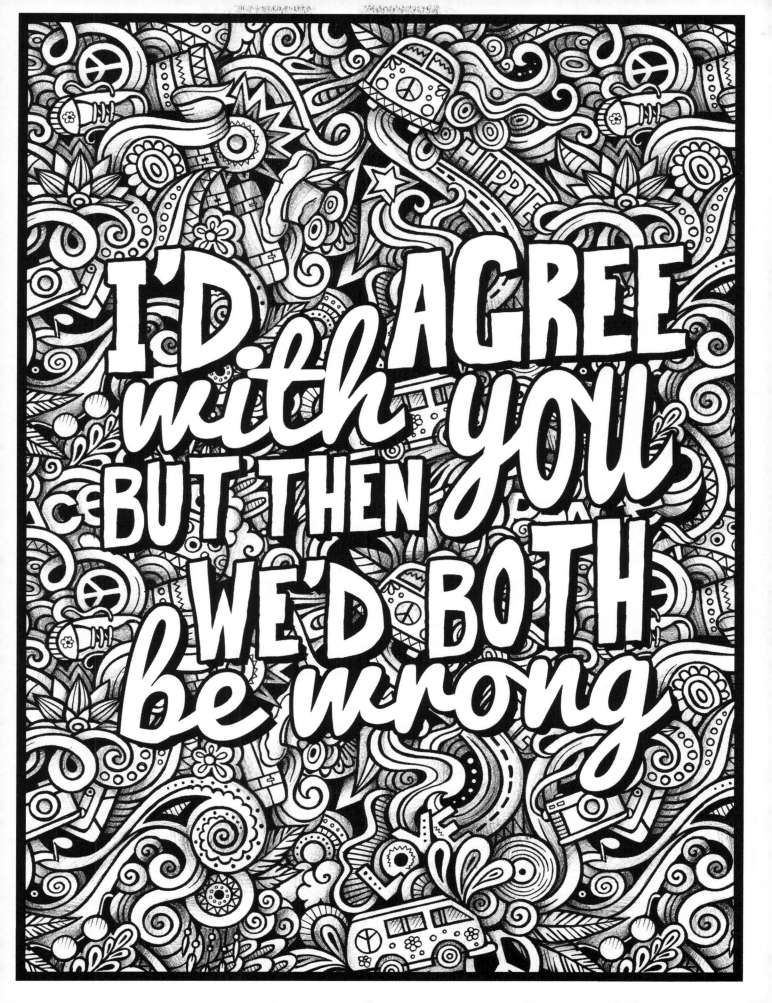

SORRY, BUT YOUR PASSWORD MUST CONTAIN A SYMBOL. A NUMBER. AN UPPERCASE LETTER. A HIEROGLYPH A HAIKU and THE BLOOD of a VIRGIN

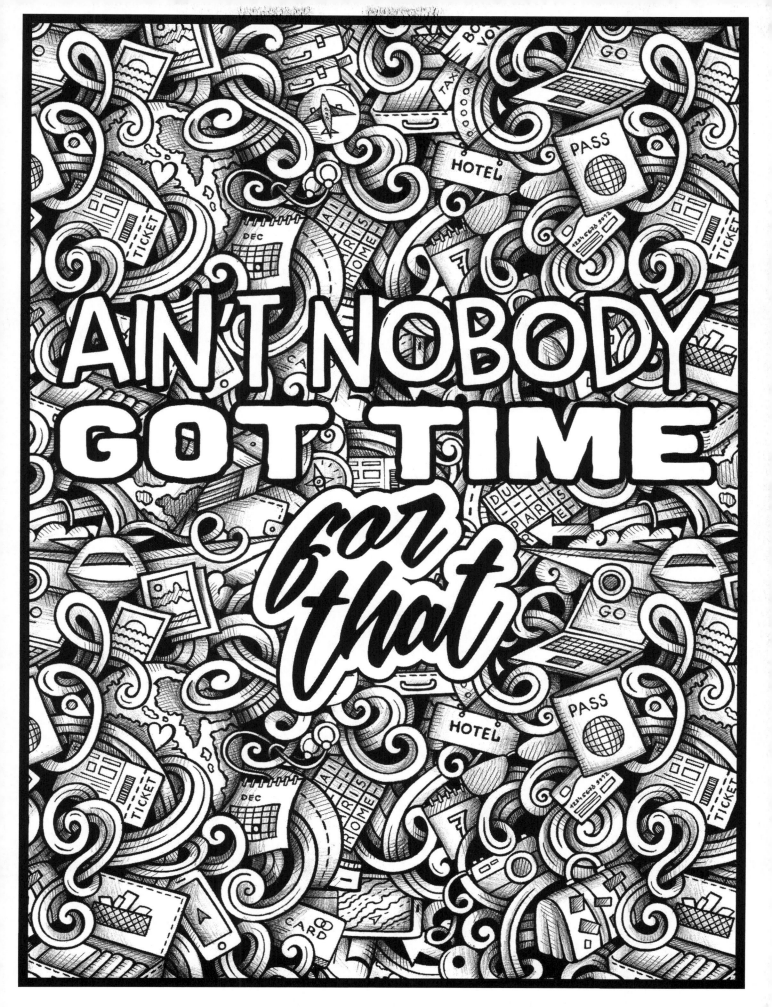

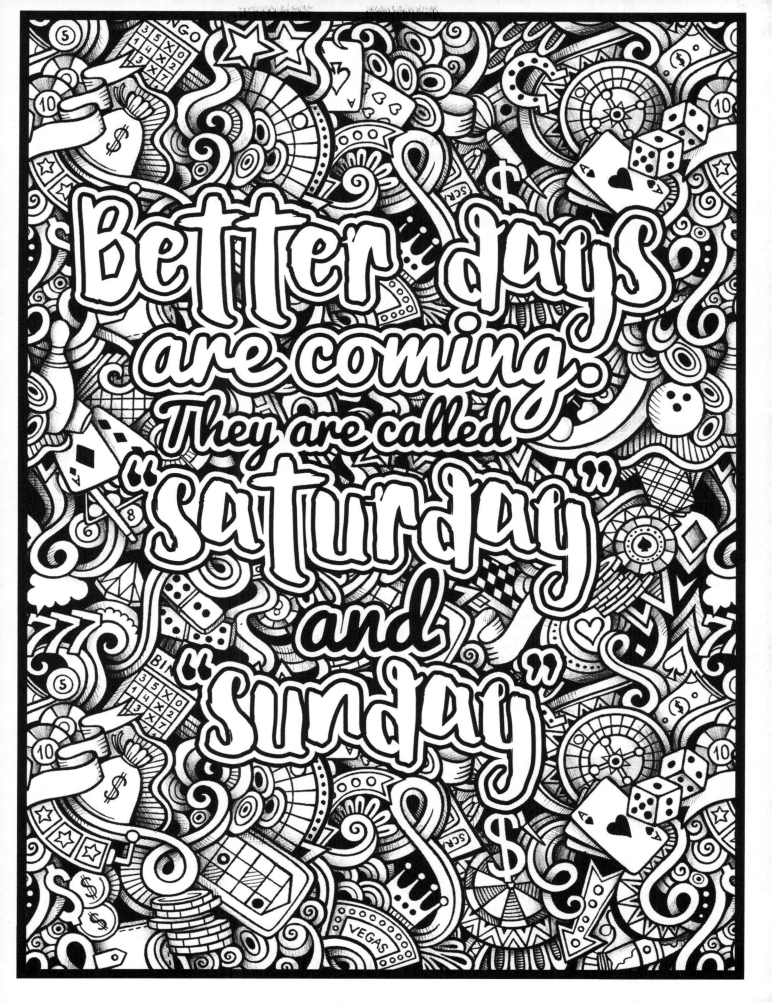

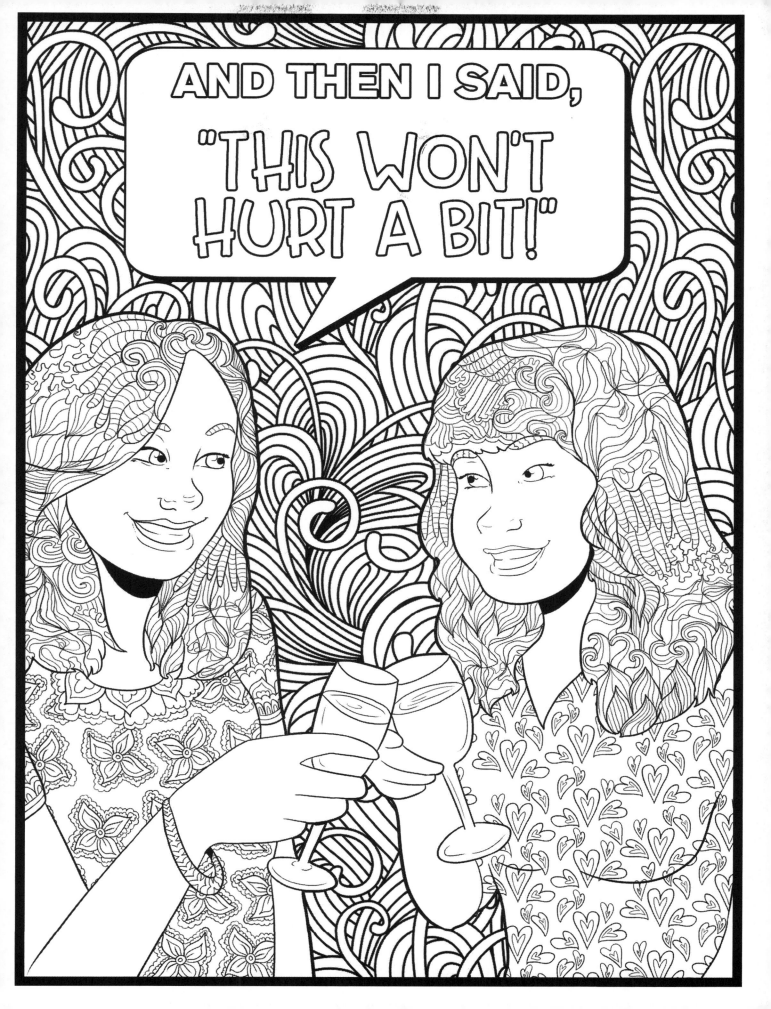

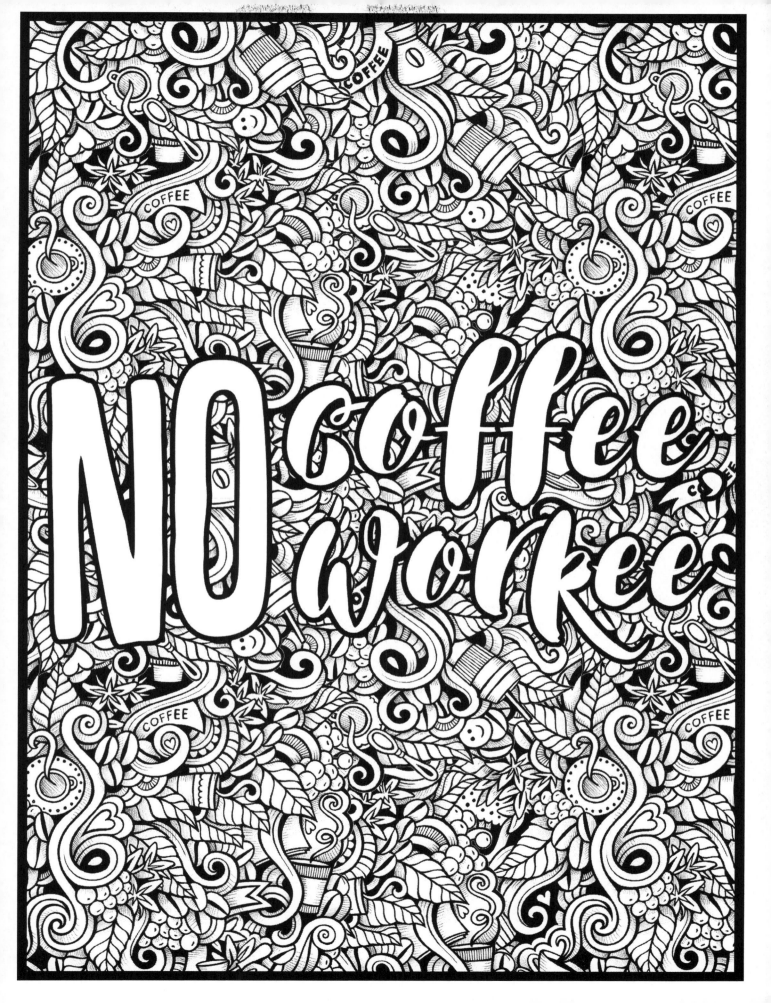

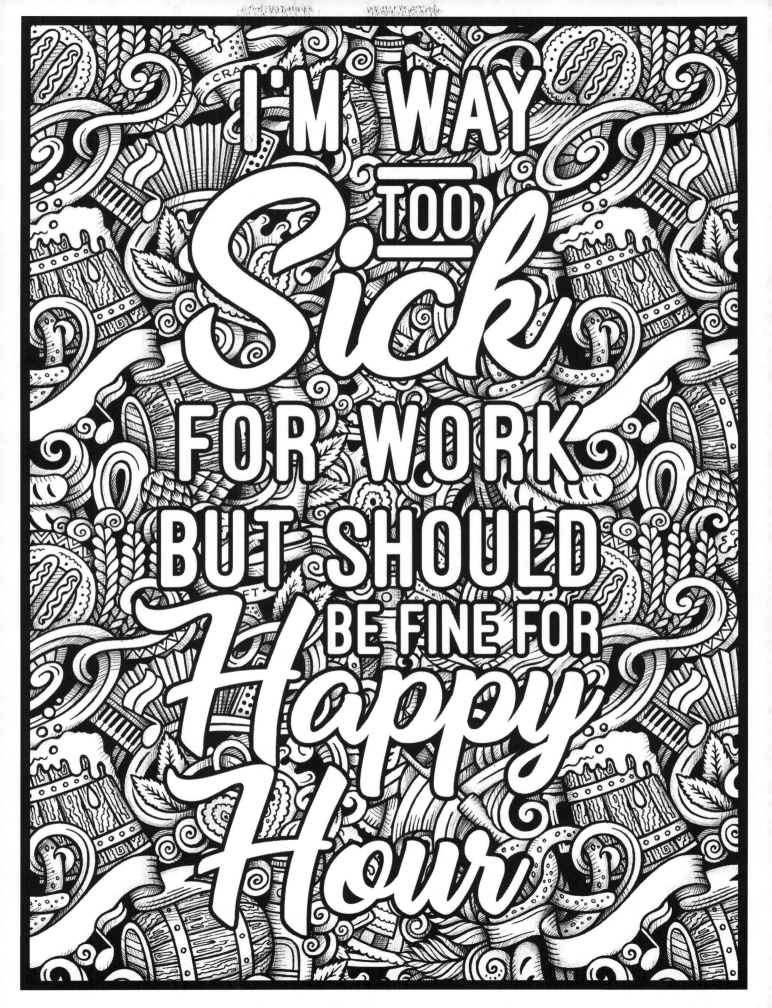

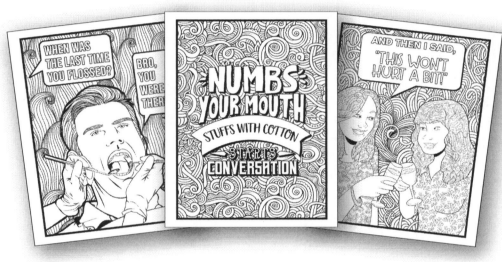
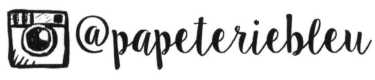
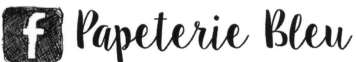

Want free goodies?
Email us at freebies@pbleu.com

@papeteriebleu

Papeterie Bleu

Shop our other books at
www.pbleu.com

Wholesale distribution through Ingram Content Group
www.ingramcontent.com/publishers/distribution/wholesale

For questions and customer service, email us at
support@pbleu.com

Printed in Great Britain
by Amazon